The Suppers Programs
Facilitator Manual

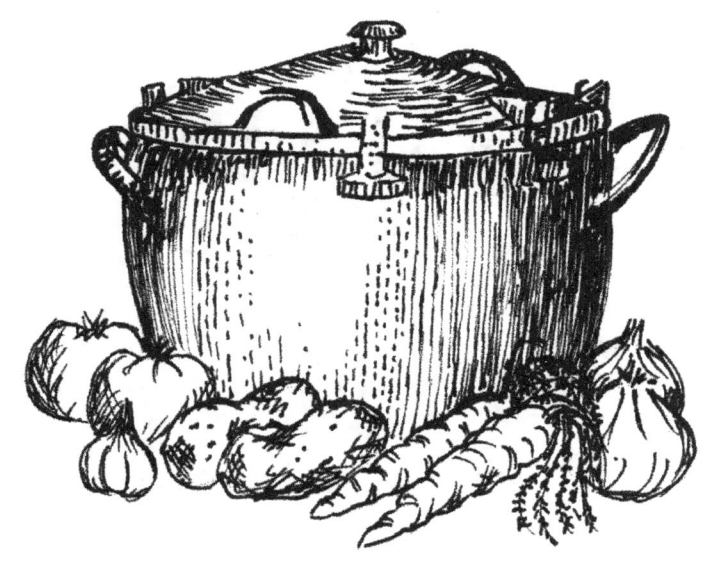

"If you can make a pot of coffee, you can make a pot of soup."

www.TheSuppersPrograms.org

The Suppers Programs
Facilitator Manual

Contents

How to Make a Successful Suppers Meeting

Every Suppers group has a distinct personality, shaped by the priorities of the people who create it. There is no rigid formula for designing a group, nor perfect schedule for having meetings. But there are common elements shared by successful meetings. Topping the list are the facilitators. If the facilitators are gratified by the experience, they will create the right environment for learning and healing.

*For those interested in becoming a Suppers Facilitator, see the Appendix for a roadmap towards qualification.

Elements of a Successful Suppers Group

1. Gratified facilitators who take pleasure in the work of Suppers and understand how to create a warm and safe environment.
2. A whole food preparation component, which can include: preparing food together, bringing in food educators, bringing a potluck meal together, and/or sharing recipes.
3. Suppers literature, including the leader's script and readings from Logical Miracles that teach the boundaries and concepts and relay the core messages of: actively practicing nonjudgment, whole food preparation, avoidance of commercial messages and restoration of the family table.
4. Sufficient planning in the way of emails and phones calls, grocery shopping, set up, food prep, clean up, reimbursement and topic selection so that the work is shared and the meetings run smoothly enough.

And that's it! As long as people come together with a mutual desire to lead a healthier life, the rest is just the details.

Starting Assumptions

The starting assumption of The Suppers Programs is that if people do what they need to do to sustain normal blood sugar and mood chemistry, their other diet and lifestyle challenges will fall into place. We focus on normalizing blood sugar and mood chemistry because your body provides very clear signals about how it is responding to food and circumstances, and you can learn to read these signals. Understanding how you feel relative to what your blood sugar and mood chemistry are doing may help you feel motivated to make healthy change. Our beginner questionnaire (page 61) and the blood sugar/mood chemistry chart of feelings (page 73) can help people determine if eating processed food is creating problems for them.

This entire document is available electronically as a PDF so you can print handouts. Go to www.TheSuppersPrograms.org

---

Suggested Leader's Script

Please take a breath . . . and join us in the opening:
Let gratitude fill me
Family and friendship sustain me
And respect for my body, mind, and spirit
Guide my choices.

Welcome to the tables of Suppers. Suppers is a learn-by-doing program for people who want more vibrant health. All you need to join is the willingness to start making diet and lifestyle changes. The program is based on whole-food preparation, restoration of family tables, and formation of healthy habits that, though simple, are hard to follow without support. At Suppers, we don't tell you what or how to eat. Our focus is on supporting your personal pathway to better health using whole food. You set the course and the pace. While you're at the Suppers table, you'll receive unconditional support, regardless of the pace of your progress. At Suppers, we're committed to the active practice of nonjudgment because we know people don't heal when they feel judged.

The only requirement for membership is the desire to lead a healthier life. The only fee you will ever pay is the shared cost of the meal.

The only investment you will ever make is your own time and effort, and the payoff is more vibrant health for you, your loved ones, and anyone to whom you pass on the program. What we ask in return is that all who attend embrace our nonprofit spirit and share their experience while refraining from the promotion of any particular diet, product, or service.

The meal comes to about $_____ today; did everyone remember to reimburse the kitty?

(*Read only if we have newcomers.*) We have a newcomer today so let's go once around the table without comment or questions, introduce ourselves by first name, and briefly share what brings us to Suppers.

Are there any announcements?

To familiarize you with our program, we read a boundary at each meeting and a passage from our literature. Today I have selected:

Boundary #_____ and _____

Welcome to the tables of Suppers!

(Eat and Meet)

Closing:
Thank you for joining our family table, for offering your friendship, and sharing your self. Our parting wish for you is that you find the healthier life you seek in body, mind, and spirit.

The Suppers Programs
Participant Questionnaire

You may participate fully in The Suppers Programs whether or not you complete this questionnaire.

First Name Only _____ Today's Date _____

Email:

In which Suppers Programs are you participating? _____ Day _____

Who else will be served by your participation? (Ex. children, diabetic mother)

Please comment on your reasons for participating:

____ I experience some of the problems or symptoms associated with low blood sugar or poor mood chemistry (depression, anxiety, fatigue, cravings, poor sleep, addictive feelings, crankiness, poor concentration, impatience).
Other: _____
____ Someone close to me experiences some of the problems or symptoms associated with low blood sugar or poor mood chemistry.
Which symptoms: _____
____ I have a professional interest.
____ I want to support my recovery from _____.
____ I am concerned for my children.
____ These problems run in my family.
____ I would like to be less dependent on medications.
____ I have come to support others, mentor and/or facilitate.
____ Emotional support.
____ Support learning how to make diet and lifestyle changes.
____ Weight loss.
____ Other: _____

Knowing that the Suppers mission is to provide safe and friendly settings where anyone – and especially people with food-related health challenges – can develop and manage their personal transition to a healthier life, how would you state your goal(s)?

Place your email here _____ if you would like us to send you instructions for joining our PRIVATE Facebook page, where we support each other and share whole food-based photos, recipes, and tips. We ask questions and advise about Suppers events (which do sometimes involve commercial relationships). Administrators remove commercial messages, limit political messages, and discourage posts not related to better health through diet and lifestyle change based on whole food.

Welcome to Suppers (for Newcomers)

Before you start your first meeting, please take a moment to learn about what you can expect. Please take home brochures and handouts, which are free.

The first part of the meeting is about preparing delicious meals of whole foods. There is no fee; you just reimburse the facilitator for the shared cost of the meal. If you don't already know how to prepare food, we'll teach you; you just jump in and start anywhere. Over time, you'll pick up the skills as you learn by watching and doing and attend special meetings with cooking mentors, if you want to.

The second part is eating and meeting. You can expect lively and informative discussions at the table, all related to healing through diet and lifestyle change. We ask that you help us keep it to one conversation going at a time; it's a way of honoring that Suppers is not a club, it's a program for people who gather with a mutual purpose in mind. You can expect that the facilitator and other members will protect the safety, warmth, and camaraderie of our environment and:

- make sure anyone who wants to share has the opportunity to do so
- guide the discussion away from promotional messages in case anyone slips into promotion of a particular diet, product or service
- preserve the atmosphere of nonjudgment, the primary requirement for helping the greatest number of people to heal
- require hand washing with soapy water after handling money or coughing

There are also a few things we will expect from you as you learn to work The Suppers Programs. We need you to:

- RSVP and come on time with small bills to pay for your meal
- preserve the safety, warmth and camaraderie of our meetings by respecting members' anonymity, using first names only and not mentioning to people outside the meeting whom you saw and what they said
- avoid using perfumes and scents at meetings as so many of us have allergies
- wash your hands before working in the kitchen or any time you cough or otherwise contaminate your hands (we have many members with special concerns for their immune systems)
- refrain from the promotion of any particular diet, product, or service
- conduct yourself in a way that preserves the safety, warmth, and camaraderie of the at-home meeting environment and honors the privilege of being invited into someone's personal space

We do not expect that you will love our food the first day or change your habits overnight. We will support you for as long as it takes you to do your own food experiments and observations and explore the many possible pathways to a healthier life.

Boundaries for Relationships

Twelve boundaries define our roles and protect the members, spirit, and culture of the Suppers groups. Observing these boundaries helps members keep the focus on their own path to wellness, allowing each of us to determine our own way using the authentic settings of the Suppers tables and the real settings of life.

1. The only requirement for membership is the desire to lead a healthier life.

2. Members actively practice nonjudgment for the sake of self, others, and group health. We foster a spirit of curiosity and experimentation to assure healing for the greatest number.

3. Suppers embraces the time-honored tradition of anonymity, using first names only. Attendance at Suppers constitutes commitment to refrain from the mention of what is said and who is seen at meetings.

4. Our only food bias is that in favor of whole food. Omnivores, vegans, and vegetarians are all served by Suppers, though individual meetings may be set up based on dietary preferences.

5. The only fee is the cost to cover groceries and any fee associated with the location. Suppers meetings refrain from profit-making relationships. Members neither pay for services nor promote commercial interests. Each Suppers group is self-supporting. Outside speakers and literature are welcome. In the spirit of curiosity and experimentation, the Suppers forum invites educational but not promotional messages.

6. The role of the facilitator is to gently guide meetings according to the agreed-upon format, concepts, and boundaries of the group. Facilitators help members honor each other's competence to determine their own paths, model nonjudgment, and protect the emotional safety of the environment. Facilitators do not give advice on matters of health; rather, they help members create experiments and observe their own experiences.

7. The role of members is to honor each other's competence and determine for themselves the path they'll each take to a healthier life. The steps will include listening, experimenting, self-observing, sharing if they care to, and deciding their course for themselves. Members honor each other's personal and emotional space and respect the privilege of being invited into someone else's home by observing house rules.

8. The role of therapeutic friends is to provide support to each other on an as-needed basis as cooking mentors, walking partners, willing ears, and supporters of those who are journaling or doing Suppers experiments.

9. At Suppers we do not recognize experts. We value expertise and especially the sharing of experiences but refrain from elevating even well researched personal biases. This boundary helps us keep the focus on biological individuality and the competence of each member to choose his or her own path to a healthier life.

10. Each group is autonomous, co-created by its members, and has its own personality. Details such as type of meeting, time, format options, food budget, RSVPs, and food preferences are up to its members. At general Suppers meetings, there is broad tolerance of dietary preferences. The only bias is that in favor of whole food.

11. Suppers meetings are no substitute for therapy or treatment. Suppers is about support for diet and lifestyle changes. Members take responsibility for getting professional help as needed.

12. We orient ourselves to service in the wider world by modeling behaviors of nonjudgment and healthy living, as we understand it.

Stories that Teach Boundaries

Boundary 1: The Only Requirement for Membership is the Desire to Lead a Healthier Life

Taylor's Story: My Primary Relationship

It is not lost on me that the first boundary for relationships at Suppers is about my relationship with myself. "The only requirement for membership is the desire to lead a healthier life" is a boundary that challenges me to examine my motivation. In the past, my health was not something I thought much about. I never considered the health benefits or deficits associated with anything I put in my mouth. I didn't question the health implications of different modes of transportation, and if I played a sport it was for fun and diversion, not because of some abstract thing called "health."

But "health" isn't so abstract any more. My belly is tangible, my joints speak to me, and my doctor is in my face with questions. *Do I want to be healthier?* Yes. *Why?* Because being unhealthy is inconvenient and uncomfortable. *Do I want to lead a healthier life?* That's a different question. That sounds like work, not desire! I associate desire with dessert, love, or a good massage.

The desire to lead a healthier life has been thrust on me by the consequences of many years of unhealthy living. My body's aches and pains brought me to Suppers; easing my physical symptoms will have to suffice as motivation until relief becomes desire for more right living.

Discussion
Consider what motivates you to lead a healthier life.

Boundary 2: Nonjudgment

Members actively practice nonjudgment for the sake of self, others, and group health. We foster a spirit of curiosity and experimentation to assure healing for the greatest number.

Libby's Story: Libby the Guinea Pig

For me, the most meaningful words from the Suppers literature appear in the second boundary for relationships: "We foster a spirit of curiosity and experimentation to assure healing for the greatest number." How refreshing! How utterly different from anything I've ever experienced. How empowering to look to my own body for data. I didn't know I was a wealth of information. But I am!

I was such a prisoner of my own thinking that it never occurred to me that I could test my blood sugar more than twice a day. The insurance company covered only two strips per day, and that was that. With my newfound fascination for my body, I bought extra strips and blasted through them for a few weeks to see how my body reacted to specific foods, exercise, and stressors. "Know your numbers" became my new motto.

I counted carbs and fiber and wrote down everything I ate and how it made me feel in my journal.

I did the breakfast challenge. That was eye opening! The oatmeal and apple that had been recommended didn't carry me nearly as long as a bowl of lentil soup or an omelet. I can't believe that I can eat in such a way that I'm not troubled by hunger pangs by 10:30. But I can.

As I got more sophisticated about my experiments, I branched into other areas of my life. I've always refused to take drugs for my insomnia, but I was willing to manipulate all kinds of behaviors to see what could help me sleep. Eating earlier helped. Making myself stay up doing needlepoint until 11:30 meant I got my sleep in one block, instead of two blocks separated by three fretful hours in the middle of the night. I played with the timing of my supplements and took notes. I took the clock out of my room.

I got curious about relationships too. I wondered what would happen if I did something totally new and out of character. The next time I felt criticized by my office mate, instead of staying in my pattern and getting defensive, I agreed with her. "You might be right," became my new reply. I got so smooth nobody could lock horns with me any more and I felt clever and happier.

Curiosity can be a gentle way of walking through life. I'm less stressed. I'm more fun. And nobody has to be down for me to be up. I love being a guinea pig, as long as I'm the one designing the experiments.

Discussion
Share what you are learning from experiments with lifestyle change.

Boundary 3: Anonymity

Suppers embraces the time-honored tradition of anonymity, using first names only. Attendance at Suppers constitutes commitment to refrain from the mention of what is said and who is seen at meetings.

Leah's Story: Anonymity

I froze when I got to my first Suppers meeting and saw a co-worker standing at the counter squeezing lemons. She looked at me blankly for a second, and then smiled broadly. "Welcome to Suppers," she said. Flashing through my mind were all the things I would not be able to talk about now because someone who works for the same company would be listening: the depression that plagues me, my sense of enslavement to certain foods, and the job stress that makes it all worse. But she was smiling, so she obviously knew something I didn't know.

What she knew was that Suppers has torn a page out of the 12-step process, using first names only and requiring members to refrain from the mention of what is said and who is seen at meetings. My colleague volunteered to sit down with me and go over the newcomer's welcome. She disclosed a few vulnerabilities of her own, which made it possible for me to start sharing my concerns right at my first meeting. Funnily enough, the two of us have been juggling a lot of the same issues with food. I would never have known this to look at her; she always seems so together. And she thought the same of me.

Without a boundary for relationships that protects anonymity, I would not be able to participate in Suppers. The shame is too deep and the pain is too raw. But with that boundary in place, not only do I eat once a week among people who really know me, I have a friend at work who meets me weekdays at the salad bar.

Discussion
What does the third boundary – anonymity – give you?

Boundary 4: Whole Food

Our only food bias is that in favor of whole food. Omnivores, vegans, and vegetarians are all served by Suppers, though individual meetings may be set up based on dietary preferences.

Gabrielle's Story: Our Only Food Bias

Our Monday Suppers meeting is a little chaotic and very fun. It's not organized around any particular diagnosis or issue, it's just a bunch of people who want to learn to prepare healthy food and forge relationships with others who want to do the same. We invite presenters to teach us how to use equipment or prepare particular cuisines; sometimes we have guest speakers. This general meeting attracts people with a range of different food preferences and strong (not to mention incompatible) ideas about what "healthy" food is.

I don't know how we manage, but we do. Suppers is not about any particular diet, but we do adhere to the basic assumption that the healthiest food is food that's as close as possible to how it occurs in nature. Whole food. One of the tricks at our particular meeting is to find recipes that are easy to adapt for vegetarians and omnivores. It makes it easy to not be critical of each other's dietary biases if we all have delicious food on our plates.

Here's what we do at the Monday lunch meeting to accommodate both vegetarians and omnivores:

1. We always have an ample, gorgeous salad, and often a fresh salsa too. Just about everybody feels well on our slaws, fresh salsas, and chopped salads.
2. We usually have a soup, stew, or chili that is suitable for vegetarians, and then add the meat to a separate pot.
3. We divvy up the price of groceries based on the menu, which is only fair because fish and meat usually increase the food costs and the vegetarians shouldn't have to cover our costs.
4. We do book reports and presentations, being careful to use "I-statements" so that it's clear we're talking about our preferences, not imposing our biases on others.
5. Some of us attend other meetings where everyone comes together to learn vegetarian food preparation. In The Suppers Programs our only food bias is that in favor of whole food, though individual meetings may form around shared dietary preferences.

Discussion
Talk about the food you think is healthiest for you and remember to use "I-statements" and avoid promoting any particular diet.

Gabrielle's Collards and Black-eyed Pea Stew
(Vegan and meat versions)

Ingredients
1 large onion, diced
2 ribs celery, chopped
1 yellow pepper, diced
4 cloves garlic, chopped fine

Olive oil to coat the pan
1 lb black-eyed peas, cooked ahead according to package directions
2 tsp Italian seasoning
1 bunch collard greens, chopped
1 16-oz can fire-roasted tomatoes (or fresh in season)
4 cups water
4 tsp organic vegetable soup base
¼ tsp cayenne
½ tsp paprika
2 TBS tomato paste
Hot sauce to taste
May or may not need a little salt

Directions
Coat the bottom of the pan with olive oil and sauté the onions until they start to brown.
Add the celery, pepper, and garlic and sauté for a few minutes.
Add the black-eyed peas and remaining ingredients and enough water to cover the beans plus ½ inch. Stir in the soup base.
Simmer about 20 minutes or until greens are soft enough, adding water as needed to make a thick stew.

Optional: 4 sausages, steamed and browned in a little oil. Cut into discs and combine with the soup after the vegetarians have been served. We used organic lamb sausage.

Serves about 8.

Gabrielle's Grapefruit Salsa

Ingredients
3 pink grapefruits, peeled, seeded, and cut in chunks
1 red pepper, diced
1 burpless cucumber, diced
1 small red onion, diced
Optional: chopped cilantro (can be passed at the table)

Dressing
About ¼ cup olive oil
A generous amount of ground black pepper, about ½ tsp
¼ tsp sea salt

Directions
Combine the fruit and vegetables in an attractive bowl.
Add the oil, salt, and pepper and combine well.
We served this with plain baked salmon.

Makes 10 servings.

14

Boundary 5: No Commercial Interests

The only fee is the cost of groceries. Suppers meetings refrain from profit-making relationships, neither paying for services nor promoting commercial interests. Each Suppers group is self-supporting, raising only enough money to cover the meeting costs of groceries and location. Outside speakers and literature are welcome. In the spirit of curiosity and experimentation, the Suppers forum invites educational but not promotional messages.

Francesca's Story: Empowered to Experiment

One of the things I like best about shopping in the produce section of our local organic food store is that there are no visual assaults. No packages with lists of ingredients, no health claims, no plastic signs helping me make my decisions based on someone else's profit motive. The only messages are little paper signs telling me how many miles it took to bring each item to market. Bin after bin, red, orange, green, the vegetables and fruits are perfectly fresh if not perfectly formed. No buckets of golf ball perfect plums or tennis ball oranges, no waxed, flawless, tasteless (sprayed) Frankenapples. Real food.

Sometimes I leave Suppers and go straight to the health food store so I can reinforce what I learned at lunch by preparing my family's dinner. Following a discussion of the fifth boundary and the spirit of experimentation, I did just that. For too long, I have been an uncreative, uninspired, reluctant cook. No wonder my kids and husband went for the packaged stuff, it was the only food in the house that had any flavor.

No more. At my Suppers meeting, the emphasis is mostly on learning to make healthy, delicious food. So the aspect of the program related to reversing diseases doesn't apply to me. It's more about prevention, rejoicing in natural foods, and building a community around mutual interest in good food. What's been most liberating for me is feeling empowered to experiment with flavor and learn from cooks and chefs who donate their time to teach at Suppers meetings.

Removing the profit motive and keeping the focus on educational messages has made it possible for many of us to participate who otherwise could not afford to learn how to prepare beautiful healthy food. The Suppers culture of experimentation has freed me to create. I have a new toolbox at home, and I got all the tools from the local whole food store.

Here is what it contains:

> Cilantro and citrus fruits: turn any meat, fish, fowl, or bean dish into a zesty treat in 10 minutes with a fresh salsa made with almost any fruits.
> Coconut fat for healthier, more delicious frying.
> My own herbed rubbing salt, fragrant with cardamom. (see page 16)
> Nuts to chop and pan toast with a little olive oil and fresh parsley to top anything savory.
> White, golden balsamic, or coconut vinegar for quick dressings that light up a shredded cabbage or beet slaw in seconds.
> Kale, collards, or spinach to shred and add last minute to soup, stew, or chili, as much for their brilliant emerald green as for the health benefits they bestow.

And last but not least, I now have a new little garden patch outside my kitchen where chives, sorrel, thyme, basil, and parsley are waiting for me to come up with a new, liberating flavor experiment.

So many of my family's basic human needs are taken care of simultaneously as I do all the little things it takes to gather us around a table of colorful food.

Discussion
How do you benefit from learning in an environment without commercial messages?

Francesca's Seasoning Salt

Ingredients
3 TBS coarse salt (we use Himalayan or Celtic)
¼ tsp cayenne pepper (or paprika, if you don't want the heat)
½ tsp ground cardamom (fresh crushed seed is best, if you can get it)
1 tsp ground pepper

Directions
Combine the ingredients and keep on hand in a glass jar.

Amaranth Cakes

Ingredients
1 cup amaranth
2 cups water
Salt to taste
1 tsp onion powder
Coconut fat for frying

Directions
Place the amaranth in a hot saucepan. Cook dry while stirring constantly until the grains begin to turn golden and you hear lots of popping.
Add the water, salt, and onion powder and whisk to get out the lumps of onion powder.
Turn heat to low and simmer for 15 minutes or until done, stirring as needed. Cool.
Heat enough coconut fat to cover the skillet.
Form the amaranth porridge into small cakes and place in the hot oil.
Fry until deep golden brown on both sides and serve immediately.
If they stick to the pan, they probably aren't done. Letting them cook a bit longer will usually solve the problem.

Serves 8 – 12

Make Your Own Fruit Salsa Recipe

Ingredients
½ bunch cilantro
1 red pepper, finely diced
Juice of 1 lime and 1 orange
Pinch of salt
Drizzle of olive oil
6 cups of diced fruit like plums, mangos, or apples

Directions
Combine the ingredients. If using a fruit like apples that brown quickly once cut, toss them with the citrus juices as you dice them.

Optional: 2 minced jalapeno peppers

Makes about 12 servings.

Boundary 6: Facilitator's Role

The role of the facilitator is to gently guide meetings according to the agreed-upon format, concepts, and boundaries of the group. Facilitators help members honor each other's competence to determine their own path, model nonjudgment, and protect the emotional safety of the environment. Facilitators do not give advice on matters of health; rather, they help members create experiments and observe their own experiences.

Andrea's Story: Relationship Service

Fortunately I'd been attending Suppers meetings for a while and knew what to expect. When the discussion drifted into turbulent waters, I knew that the facilitator would draw us back into a safe setting – this is the facilitator's number one responsibility.

The subject on the table was "relationship services," the little things we do each day for our family and friends. It is a topic that makes many of us uncomfortable and/or critical of others. At our table was a mixed group of mostly women, some of whom had decided to stay home and raise their children, some who had gone back to work full time, and some who thought part time work was right for them while they had small children at home. This was a charged topic for me because I'm living in the tension of these decisions right now.

I could feel my temperature rise as someone wondered "Why do people bother to have children if they aren't going to spend time with them." It was all I could do to not yell at her, "If I don't work, we don't eat!" when the facilitator intervened. "Whoa," she said. "I need us all to take a breath and remember we're at Suppers. Let's each talk about our own experience."

We are obliged by the culture of the Suppers setting to actively work at not judging, to honor the competence of each member to find his or her own path to a healthier life. Part of this is navigating through uncomfortable feelings and keeping the focus on ourselves. It means refraining from criticisms that may bring us momentary relief but compromise the feel of the group. There are some things we each have to muddle through ourselves. And how to balance self-care, caring for family, and the economic necessity to produce income is one of them.

I think reactivity is the confounder of digestion. It is a ruiner of relationships. Here was an opportunity to observe that balancing home life and work life is thorny, and share how we cope. Without judging anyone else's way of coping, we were able to go around the table and each name one of our "best practices."

The facilitator started:
"I eat in such a way that my blood sugar and mood chemistry are not what's driving my mood and how I relate to people at home and at work."

"I call my husband and ask him to chop the vegetables. The biggest thing that gets in the way of my serving healthy meals is that endless chopping."
"I get to a meeting once a week; it's one small thing I can do to take care of myself."

"I go to the door when my husband gets home and look him straight in the eyes and tell him I'm happy to see him. That 20 seconds brings huge dividends throughout the evening."

"I make dinner every night and have the kids come help with prep, even if only for 10 minutes. I want them to assume that they are going to be doing this as adults."

And the one dad who was there said:

"No matter what else is going on, if I'm in town, bedtime stories are my job. And I agree, the small investment bears huge dividends."

I could not work on the health issue that brought me to meetings if I couldn't depend on the Suppers cultural commitment to provide safe settings. The use of "I-statements," the group intention to achieve healing for the greatest number, and the commitment to social behavior that promotes digestion are all just as important as developing a taste for foods that normalize my blood sugar.

Discussion
Name a relationship service you enjoy giving and one you like to receive.

Boundary 7: Member's Role

The role of members is to honor each other's competence and determine for themselves the path they'll each take to a healthier life. The steps will include listening, experimenting, self-observing, sharing if they care to, and deciding their course for themselves. Members honor each other's personal and emotional space and respect the privilege of being invited into someone's home by observing house rules.

Gina's Story: The Role of Members

I am torn between wishing there were more men at meetings and then not feeling comfortable sharing when men do come to meetings. There are all kinds of things I don't want to share in mixed company, and breast cancer is one of them. I have arrived at an age when my friends are starting to get diagnosed.

But there I was at Suppers, where I'm supposed to be working on my listening skills and honoring everyone's personal and emotional space. So when the subject came up at a meeting one night and there were a couple of men there, I had one of those growth opportunities that are so uncomfortable. I have to give the men credit for showing up after a long day at work (why I need to give them more credit than I give the working women, I don't know). One of them said, "Everything I know about breast cancer I learned from a man." He had a good friend whose wife had been treated for it. What blew me away was that this man knew more about tumors and nodes and centimeters and radiation and chemo and herbs and medications than I did. For him to have known all that, he must have had some very intimate conversations with his friend, and his friend must have been willing to share some very personal details. This man spoke with such compassion for his friends that it blew all my prejudices about how men communicate right out of the water.

I decided that very night how I was going to work at being a better member of a group. I had two goals: to be more present in my listening and to be more real in my sharing. Even if a man talks in more typical guy fashion, I can listen to the content and stop judging the delivery.

Properly executing my role as a member of a group is important because the quality of the job I do determines the benefits I receive.

Discussion
Describe the personal pathway to better health you are designing. How do actively practicing nonjudgment and knowing you will not be judged play a role?

Boundary 8: Therapeutic Friendship

The role of therapeutic friends is to provide support to each other on an as-needed basis, as cooking mentors, walking partners, willing ears, and supporters of those who are journaling or doing Suppers experiments.

Simone's Story: Therapeutic Friendship

If there's one thing I've learned in recovery it's that I have a disease of disconnection. Even though I'm not the best connector, I know I need the support of other people, especially when I'm making uncomfortable but necessary changes. For a while, my identity hinged on the not doing of something – not drinking. I celebrated one-week, one-month, one-year anniversaries of not drinking. While there was considerable satisfaction in these milestones, I felt bad that so much of my energy went into the *not doing* of something.

When I heard there was a program that promoted healthy eating so people could feel more comfortable in their bodies, I knew exactly what they meant. Although I was done with alcohol, I was still always searching for the next little fix, food, sex, or thrill of any kind. But after the rise there was always the crash.

At Suppers I have been taken under wing by a community of "food sleuths." The members form therapeutic friendships based on helping each other get their needs met so their bodies can heal. This is how we do service. In my case, the help I needed most was finding out which foods were my worst triggers for craving baked goods and which foods put me in a quiet good mood (square meals, like roasted turkey, yams, and greens). I also needed help getting over feeling sorry for myself because I did go through a period of feeling deprived.

Suppers doesn't ask much of me. The clearest, easiest thing I can give to the program is provide friendship services and support the growing population of people who look to their diet and lifestyle for solutions.

Discussion
Imagine that you are already getting the support you need to support healthy change. Who is doing what?

Boundary 9: No Experts

At Suppers we do not recognize experts. We value expertise and especially the sharing of experiences but refrain from elevating even well researched personal biases. This boundary helps us keep the focus on biological individuality and the competence of each member to choose his or her own path to a healthier life.

Mary Ellen's Story: Sacred Cows

If they asked for a poster child for dietary solutions to mental health problems, I would volunteer. I'm a passionate advocate of nutritional psychology, because I got off antidepressants easily once I started eating well. But I have to be careful how I talk at meetings. The topic on the table was the ninth boundary, which reminds us to value expertise without elevating even well researched biases to the status of truth. It was a lively conversation, to put it mildly. We had people who felt they owed their lives to their nutritionists and doctors and others who had had very bad experiences. Personally, I had been on and off hormone replacement therapy, on and off medicine for bone health, shifting around as Medicine changed its mind about how to handle women's bones after menopause. There was an anti-vaccine advocate and several of us who can't believe anybody would be against vaccinating. It was one of those days when we all had to work at nonjudgment. We were drawn into a discussion of fallen "sacred cows" or medical ideas that had once been gospel and then fallen into disfavor.

"It's medical gospel until it's not." One member's mental health issues finally cleared up after an alternative therapy to detox heavy metals. She was particularly skeptical. "They thought I was cuckoo until they found the explanation. Then I was just a patient with some very specific work to do.

The people in my Suppers group are readers. It seemed everybody was aware of some test, nutrient or procedure that, while once gospel, had fallen out of favor: mammograms, which may help detect a deadly but small risk of preventable death but might also lead to surgery for something that would never become a threat. Hormone replacement therapy, the fountain of youth until they realized it might cause stroke and heart attacks. Arthroscopic surgery: one day yes, the next day no. Low fat is good; oops, no, it's bad. They still can't make up their minds about that one. Eggs are the enemy; no, eggs are the perfect health food. Cholesterol-lowering drugs are good; oh dear, maybe their side effects are not. Take calcium; well, no, not just calcium. It won't help without vitamin D. But uh oh, now we're taking too much Vitamin D. Don't eat beef. Do eat beef, but not any beef – only grass-fed. Take this drug to prevent osteoporosis. Yikes, it seems to be causing fractures!

It's a challenge in this age of information to know which experts to pay attention to. I have a lot of respect for my doctor and the vaccination program, but considering how much disease is preventable through lifestyle, I have come to a very specific conclusion. I do not want to be the lab rat. My personal expert tells me my surest path to a healthier life is prevention. And for me that includes returning to a diet and lifestyle that – as much as possible – predates all these epidemics. I will eat food as close as possible to how it occurs in nature. I will move. And I will cultivate relationships that make me feel warm and connected.

Discussion
Practice making "I-statements" and share a personal truth about healthy living. (Example: I have learned through experimenting that I feel best on a near-vegetarian diet.)

Boundary 10: Group Autonomy

Each group is autonomous, co-created by its members, and has its own personality. Details such as type of meeting, time, format options, food budget, RSVPs, and food preferences are up to its members. At general Suppers meetings, there is broad tolerance of dietary preferences. The only bias is that in favor of whole food.

Petra's Story: Group Autonomy

"Seeker" is probably the word that best describes my image of myself in recent years. Casting about for ways to explain and tame my raging mood swings has been a humbling experience. Most of the time, I'm a pretty nice, rational person. But when I snap, I'm a lunatic. Being in seeking mode has helped because it makes me feel like I'm solution oriented. As soon as I feel like I've got it all figured out, I'm more likely to slip, sugar binge, and get hostile.

Suppers helps me stay curious. It doesn't tell me what or how to eat. It encourages anyone who wants to facilitate a meeting to get creative about the goals of their particular meeting. As long as we keep the focus on using whole food, use the table experience to help people form healthy habits, and avoid commercial messages, we can get pretty creative about the details. So when I started searching for my answers, there were lots of different kinds of meetings to try. I went to general meetings, a blood sugar meeting, a farm-to-table meeting, and Living Suppers for raw vegans.

It was not an easy journey. I did lots of lying at early meetings because I was too ashamed to say I'd eaten a foot-long hot dog or a big slice of chocolate cake. What was I worried about! Nobody knew what I ate when I was at home and nobody cared. Why did I want them to think better of me? Somebody told me it didn't matter if I lied about what I ate; the program would still work.

In the end, I found I needed a hybrid of eating styles. I do absolutely the best when I eat mostly vegetables, lots of raw food, and meat only very occasionally when my body sends me a signal that it's time to have some. My sugar cravings and hostile behavior resolved together! And my sinus issues cleared up too.

Having autonomous groups makes for passionate facilitators who love teaching what they know. It means seekers like me have an array of possible eating styles to experiment with. Having options has given me a measure of control over my life and my moods that I would not have believed possible. My family has benefited as much as I have. Instead of yelling "Mom's coming, run for cover!" my kids are saying things like "What the heck is edamame?" and "Here comes the three-veg mother, pushing her vegetable obsession on everyone again." Eventually I will relax and let the kids have more say in the menu. For now I think they are just relieved to have a relatively sane person preparing their food, something I could not have accomplished without the opportunity to try different ways of eating and create the one that works for me.

Discussion

If you were to facilitate the ideal Suppers meeting for yourself, what would it be like (the menu, the population served, the handling of "housework" and details)?

Boundary 11: No Substitute for Therapy or Treatment

Suppers meetings are no substitute for therapy or treatment. Suppers is about support for diet and lifestyle changes. Members take responsibility for getting professional help as needed.

Margaret's Story: Numbers Don't Lie

A discussion of the 11th boundary helped us all make distinctions about what we could reasonably expect from a support group and what we needed to do with medical practitioners. Sometimes it's difficult for me to distinguish which issues I should be addressing with my doctor and which ones I should address on my own. I have thyroid problems and had just crossed over into type 2 diabetes at the time I started Suppers. I am conscientious about my appointments and have good relationships with the doctors who care for me. I'm also a do-it-yourselfer, and my inclination is to do everything I possibly can myself.

I did not care at all for those high fasting blood sugars. For that problem I decided to do as much as I possibly could on my own before seeking out pharmaceutical solutions.

At my Suppers meeting, nobody would tell me what changes would improve my numbers, but they did suggest experiments. To make a long story short, my self-observations revealed that if I traded most of the fruit I was eating for lentils or a small portion of meat, my numbers got better. For years I'd been eating lots of fruit because I thought it was healthy. By giving it up, I lost 10 pounds, all of it in the mid-section. My endocrinologist actually asked me what I was doing because my blood sugar normalized, my thyroid readings improved somewhat, and my triglycerides went down.

This didn't make sense to me. Fruit is health food and I love it. But numbers don't lie, and neither does my belt. After conducting several months of experiments, the conclusion I've come to is that I will deal with as many of the issues of advancing age as possible by staying curious, running experiments, and seeking solutions in my lifestyle. And when healthy change is not enough – dealing with my thyroid problem, for example – I can rely on medical practitioners and be grateful to live in a time when pharmaceutical solutions are available.

Discussion
Consider your health concerns: what can be managed with right living; what will require professional help? And what's in the gray area?

Boundary 12: Service

We orient ourselves to service in the wider world by modeling behaviors of nonjudgment and healthy living, as we understand it.

Carley's Story: Service

I am not sure which gift of working Suppers holds more meaning for me, learning to be less judgmental or learning to prepare healthy food. In a way, both things are about nourishment. The food part is obvious. But learning to not judge feeds me just as much as food because it has changed how people relate to me. The less fault finding I am in my relationships, the more people respond to me with acceptance, love, and understanding.

An important service I can provide to my group and my community is modeling healthy behaviors and attitudes. OK, to be honest there is a slight gloating feeling that goes along with having people get jealous that my children eat well and behave well, but that's only human. My behaviors reflect my pure intentions. And my intention and behaviors make people understand that I care.

I am always happy to teach people what I know, invite them to learn for themselves at Suppers, cook with their children to provide another adult role model, or listen when they need to talk about how frustrating it is to live in our society's food culture. Sometimes just listening is the greatest service I can provide.

The Suppers model of "nutritional harm reduction" is very gentle. It takes a colossal task like cleaning up the family diet and breaks it down into manageable steps that can be accomplished in no particular order. It gives people many choices about how to proceed that are doable, if not exactly easy to do. It helps people focus their energies where there is the most possibility of success instead of spinning their wheels doing the same things over and over with bad results.

Nobody rushed me along when I arrived at Suppers. Long before I acquired a taste for purifying green foods, I had to dump a load of toxic waste in the form of criticism and judgment. They kept me on a ladder looking up at some and down on others but never sharing the same space. Having received so much, it is a joyful experience for me to go forth into my community knowing there are two kinds of service I am well equipped to provide: quietly modeling nonjudgment and actively teaching others how to prepare and develop a palate for real food.

Discussion
Describe a service that has been provided to you in Suppers. Describe a service you can provide to Suppers or your community.

Concepts

These concepts are the underlying assumptions on which all of The Suppers Programs are based. We have incorporated with gratitude ideas from many fields and organizations, including environmental medicine, nutritional psychology, counseling, public health, the whole food movement, and the 12-step programs. Our literature presents a wellness orientation that emphasizes the health of the physical body and the body's role as the human terrain on which all other experience takes place. We work with the assumption that certain problems are "health relatives" because their biochemical and environmental causes are so similar. These principles apply, regardless of the diagnosis, to anyone whose health challenges require lifestyle change, including those with depression, anxiety, learning issues, obesity, diabetes, and/or problems with alcohol.

Concept 1: Biological Individuality
Every body is different from every other body

The concept of biological individuality reminds us that everyone's body is different from everyone else's body. Biological individuality is seen at all levels of health, mental health, and addictive experience. We honor each other's individuality by assuming we don't know what is right for someone else and keeping the focus first on finding our own pathways. The courage and power to change our individual biology lies in the challenging work of diet and lifestyle change. This means subtracting processed foods that light up the pleasure centers in the brain artificially and then let you crash, just as drugs do. It means adding whole foods that build stable, happy brains over time.

Concept 2: The Forgotten Body
Poor health and addiction are the logical conclusion of leaving the body out of the body, mind, and spirit equation

The Suppers Programs seek no more but no less than to restore care of the physical body to its natural place in this equation. The body's nonnegotiable needs are simple, if not easy, to fulfill. We require a diet of whole foods as they exist in nature, meaningful physical activity, and ways to manage stress, including satisfying human connections. The profit motive for orienting care of the body toward treatment and pharmaceuticals is intense. At Suppers, we remember the body and focus on prevention and repair through diet and lifestyle.

Concept 3: Food Is the First Addiction

Suppers recognizes that food is our most expensive national addiction. In human and dollar calculations, the consequences of the processed, drug-like food supply already surpass the consequences of cigarettes and alcohol. Not only does processed food lead us down the path to obesity and diabetes, the havoc wrought on blood sugar and mood chemistry sets us up for dependence on and addiction to other substances. Experts disagree on which foods have what consequences, whether or not there are good foods and bad foods, or whether there are any nutritional advantages to organic or locally grown foods. Suppers recommends we not be part of their experiment. We know that eating food as it exists in nature is safe; for everything else we are lab rats.

Concept 4: Appetite Foolishness
Desiring and repeatedly consuming things you know are hurting you

"Appetite foolishness" is characterized by craving things that are unhealthy for your body. You experience appetite foolishness if you get repeated urges to consume foods or beverages that temporarily resolve a discomfort but create a greater problem over time. Many feelings we assume are our emotions are really reactions to drug-like food. It is very easy to develop appetite foolishness in a culture that combines a food supply that is more like drugs than food with intense profit motive.

If appetite foolishness is part of your problem, the matching solution will include changes in habits. The solution is simple, but it may not be easy. It calls for 1) a diet of wholesome foods to meet personal nutritional needs, 2) new habits of mind and body, and 3) a community of family, mentors, and peers to support the change process. For some individuals, professional help will be necessary, especially when toxicity is an issue. But even the best professional help is no substitute for support from a community of caring people who want to see their loved ones thrive.

Concept 5: Automatic Choices
The choices you make when you aren't consciously participating

The concept of automatic choices tells us that if we do not consciously work on change, we will be run by our default settings or automatic choices. If appetite foolishness governs your automatic choices, you are very likely to have health, mental heath, or addiction problems. There are lots of reasons for the gaps between what we know is best and what we actually do. Here are some of the ones that drive the choices we make:

- *Unfamiliarity.* Staying the same is familiar and easy. Changing is strange and hard.
- *Discomfort.* The pain of staying the same is less than the anticipated pain of changing.
- *The nature of addiction.* The forces that make us want to change are weaker than the forces that keep us addicted.
- *Time.* Changes require intention, acquiring information, creating a plan, implementing the plan, and adjusting the plan. These things are time consuming.
- *Expectations.* We expect change to be difficult, and so it is.
- *The unknown.* The grip of addiction doesn't happen for just one reason. It's the unknown forces you aren't addressing that will sabotage your process.
- *Support.* If supports are not in place, changing and maintaining changes is sabotaged by the ease with which we can fall back into the relationship with the addiction. Appetite foolishness will prevail without support.
- *Your other personal reasons.*

You can get help from your therapeutic friends at Suppers by learning to observe how your default settings are running your life.

Concept 6: Health Relatives
People whose problems have similar biochemical and environmental causes, regardless of their diagnoses

Many people with dissimilar-sounding diagnoses are actually quite closely related because the diet and lifestyle changes needed to turn them around are virtually the same. To the extent that health problems are lifestyle-related, The Suppers Programs provide the ideal support for anyone with some combination of depression, anxiety, learning issues, obesity, diabetes, and/or problems with alcohol. These issues tend to cluster in families and individuals.

Concept 7: The Diagnosis May Be Inconsequential
If eating processed foods caused your problem to begin with, the right solution – whole food – may be more important than the diagnostic labels

Suppers welcomes people with a wide array of health and mental health challenges related to diet and lifestyle. Most of us have problems with blood sugar regulation and mood chemistry. Though nutritional requirements vary greatly from one person to the next, we all share a fundamental need for whole food. Determining which whole foods make us feel best will require doing experiments to collect the data. Suppers has nothing to do with the details of dealing with particular diagnoses; that's up to people and their practitioners. But Suppers has everything to do with providing the support people need to make health-restoring change.

Concept 8: Your Internal Observer
The part of you that notices but doesn't judge

Inside each one of us is an observer. If you ever tried meditation, you may have learned this already. It is the part of you that witnesses what you're doing while you do it or shortly after. Your internal observer is your best friend as you try to break a habit. The trick is to learn to make the observation before your internal judge takes over and charges it with uncomfortable emotions. For today, just start noticing that part of yourself that observes what you're doing while you're doing it.

Concept 9: How You Feel Is *Data*
Your body is constantly communicating important information to you, if you would just learn to interpret its language

Daytime fatigue, mental energy, depression, anxiety, cravings, mood swings, and of course good spirits, emotional stability, and freedom from impulses are all important data. You just need to learn to interpret the signals your body is sending you. At Suppers we seek to help you establish connections with the part of you that is constantly trying to send you feedback about what's going on inside and how you need to change. We do this mostly by teaching you how to do experiments and make observations about how foods and behaviors make you feel. Honoring biological individuality, Suppers does not advocate any particular diet over any other. Rather, we focus on helping people develop a palate for the freshest, healthiest whole food. Of those, Suppers experiments will help you determine which are the healthiest for you.

Concept 10: Addition and Subtraction
Good health is achieved by adding what the body needs to have and subtracting what the body needs to not have

Health challenges at the biological level boil down to two simple functions: addition and subtraction. In simplest terms, addiction, or any disease, is a combination of not having enough of something that's required for good health (deficiency) and having too much of something that is bad for health (toxicity). Whether the reasons are genetic or acquired, good biological health rests on having enough of what builds healthy cells and not having too much of what destroys cells. The task for people who are earnest about making diet and lifestyle changes for the sake of better health is to subtract the things that are making them toxic and add the things that will restore their brains and bodies to health.

Concept 11: Nutritional Harm Reduction
A gentle transition process that makes healthy change possible

People who join Suppers have at some point suffered because of the addictive nature of the food supply. With food, abstinence is not an option. That leaves harm reduction. We understand that there are many obstacles to change, particularly for those who live in households with others who are not ready to change. That's why The Suppers Programs are about reducing harm gently, supporting people as they explore their willingness to head in the direction of a healthier life. Let's face it. Are you going to eliminate everything you know is bad for you and switch to eating only things that are good for you overnight? At Suppers we see nutrition as a transitional process. It takes time to learn how to determine which foods work best for you and your family, to learn how to prepare them, and to acquire a taste for, and ultimately a desire for, healthier foods. You will probably experience all kinds of slips, relapses, and hilarious stories along the way. Self-doubt, ice-cream cones, spousal sabotage, secret eating, and rebelling children are all natural steps in the transition process. At Suppers, our stories will help you learn the many ways to reduce harm by becoming aware of automatic choices, facing appetite foolishness, experimenting with better choices and noting how you feel, and adding foods that are healthy while slowly subtracting those that are more like drugs.

Concept 12: Logical Miracle
What takes place in the natural course of things when your needs are met

The dictionary says a miracle is an extraordinary event that manifests divine intervention in the lives of humans. It is highly unusual. "Logical" simply means capable of using reason. At Suppers we assume that miracles are not so unusual after all. We can reasonably expect them to happen when people receive the nourishment and support they need in safe, nonjudgmental settings. Reversal of the progression into diabetes, freedom from food cravings, relief from depression or anxiety, and more rewarding relationships are just a few of the logical miracles we see in people who work our program. Dreams that seemed impossible prior to getting your needs met become ordinary outcomes once your needs are met. They become logical miracles.

Concept 13: Healthier Sources of Pleasure
Alternatives to food, drink, or drugs that trigger your sense of pleasure

People who have dependent relationships with any food or drink that changes how they feel are not experiencing pleasure and comfort in the ordinary, healthy way. They experience false emotions, bad and good. It's hard for people with normal wiring and biochemistry to imagine the discomfort and desperation of the person who lives in a body that can't regulate itself or get comfortable. Whether for genetic or acquired reasons, some people return over and over to food or substances that artificially stimulate the brain's pleasure centers, looking for relief from the inability to feel normal pleasure.

The concept of healthier sources of pleasure calls on us to experiment with new ways of feeling normal comfort. Eating foods that help us feel comfortable in our own skin is just one example. For some it might be socializing, dancing, or cooking with friends. This concept calls us to the family table where we can make satisfying human connections. Any relationship or group experience that helps you feel valued, understood, and connected can provide an alternative to foods and substances as a source of pleasure. At Suppers we have found creativity to be so profoundly healing that we have built opportunities to create into the flexible structure of The Suppers Programs. We have removed all profit motives; the creative energy is focused entirely on personal healing. We invite you to use our ideas, download our literature, and create your own groups.

Concept 14: Planning Is Everything
If diet and lifestyle are central to your health challenges, the solution will require lots of planning

There is no getting around the need for planning when your health demands that you change your behaviors. With the exception of type 1 diabetics, most of us at Suppers have eaten, drunk, and behaved our way into our health challenges. Environmental exposures like heavy metals and pesticides contribute too. It is so easy to slip back into familiar patterns: grabbing a slice of pizza instead of sitting down to a meal, defaulting on good intentions to exercise more, or feeling too busy to prepare a fresh salad. This is why Suppers is a program, not a club or a class. The program can only work if you work it, and that means planning: having good food ready to eat at all times, taking the initiative to buy the best fresh ingredients, making time for meaningful physical activity, and giving and getting support in a safe setting.

Concept 15: Therapeutic Friendship
The relationships that form around doing the work of Suppers

The concept of therapeutic friendship offers people the possibility of becoming the designers of their own plans for better health or recovery with the help of peers. Once we accept that each individual has a biological natural reality, the footwork is up to individuals in relationships.

The concept of therapeutic friendship calls on us to recognize wisdom, but not to identify unassailable experts at the Suppers tables or in the resources we share. Health seeking can get very frustrating when experts disagree with one another. Whose advice should we follow? In a community of therapeutic friends whose purpose is supporting healthy change, we can help each other make the best matches between our diet and lifestyle problems and our diet and lifestyle solutions.

This concept is non-hierarchical, meaning help flows both ways and all roles have value. When the teachers are ready, the students appear; and when the students are ready, the teachers appear. In a recovery community based on therapeutic friendship, individual strengths to lead or follow, learn or teach, listen or speak are equally valued.

Concept 16: The Body Is the Temple of the Soul

The spiritual foundation of The Suppers Programs is care of the physical body, the primary spiritual act. The life we experience here and now is the one we experience in our physical bodies. The addiction we experience here and now is not possible without a body. The thoughts we're thinking are influenced by the quality of our physical brains. Our spiritual experiences, thinking, attitudes, memories, emotions, joys, and traumas all take place on the terrain of the body and the cells that make it. We all have bodies. And that matters.

Concept 17: Gratitude Begets More to Be Grateful For

The Suppers Programs are grateful to all the individuals, families, programs, researchers, clinicians, and writers whose ideas give life to this program. On our web site, credit is given in "About Us," "Food," "Stories," and "Resources," as well as in our member book reviews (www.TheSuppersPrograms.org). We are grateful for experts who devote their careers to helping us and to the programs that save lives and hold answers for many of us. We are grateful for the accumulated wisdom of all who went before us, giving us more choices for our personal pathways.

Sample Menus

Beginner Menu for New Facilitators

Many of our members have had transforming experiences around eating this chili because it stabilized their blood sugar for the rest of the day, reducing anxiety symptoms. *Don't worry about precise amounts.*

Breakfast Chili for Breakfast, Lunch or Dinner

Ingredients:
2 lbs ground turkey
olive oil
 2 16-oz cans of kidney beans
1 small jar or about 1 ½ cups salsa
1 small jar tomato sauce, with no sweeteners
1 TBS chili powder
Salt, if permitted, to taste, about ½ tsp

Optional: up to 6 cups of chopped vegetables, like peppers, onion, carrots, greens

Directions:
Place enough olive oil in a soup pot to coat the bottom.
On medium heat, brown 2 lbs of ground turkey.
Add 2 cans of drained kidney or preferred beans.
Add 1 small jar of salsa and one small jar of tomato sauce.
Add optional chopped vegetables.
Depending on the amount of liquid in the salsa, you may need some water; add what you need to make it just slightly watery.
Add a tablespoon of chili powder, or to taste.
Add salt to taste, if it is not restricted for you.
Let it simmer until the water steams off a little and it is the consistency you like, about ½ hour.

Serves 8 – 12.

Serve this with a large tossed salad, figuring about 1 ½ cups of greens and veggies per person.

Tossed Salad

Ingredients:
1 head of Romaine lettuce, washed, dried and chopped
3 tomatoes, chopped
1 red onion, sliced very thin
3 carrots, chopped
2 cucumbers, chopped

2 bell peppers, chopped
1 cup Greek olives

Creamy Garlic Dressing

Ingredients:
¼ cup golden balsamic vinegar or other sweet vinegar
½ cup olive oil
½ cup organic mayonnaise
½ tsp salt
2 large cloves garlic

Optional: ¼ cup fresh herbs of choice

Directions:
Process all ingredients in the food processor until it becomes creamy.

Dresses salad for 10 – 12.

Living Suppers

Raw Walnut Pate or Non-Meatballs

Ingredients:
1 cup raw walnuts, soaked about 4 hours and drained
1 TBS lemon juice
1 tsp extra virgin olive oil
1 TBS Italian seasoning
1 tsp tamari sauce
1 clove garlic, well mashed
salt to taste, if permitted
1 TBS minced parsley
1 TBS minced onion

Directions:
Place ingredients in a food processor and pulse until pate is as fine as you want it.
Use as a spread or form into non-meatballs and serve with raw marinara sauce.

Serves 4.

Raw Marinara Sauce

Ingredients:
4 dates, pits removed
3 ripe tomatoes, seeded and chopped
½ cup oil packed sun dried tomatoes
1 red pepper, chopped
2 TBS extra virgin olive oil
¼ cup fresh basil leaves
1 tsp dried oregano
3 cloves garlic, crushed
¼ tsp salt
pepper

Directions:
Place all ingredients in the food processor and process until well blended but not pureed.

To Serve:
Serve on cooked pasta or spaghetti squash or, for a totally raw meal, serve on a bed of raw zucchini strips or spirals. Strips can be made with a vegetable peeler. Spirals can be made on a spiral slicer.

Makes sauce for about 10 servings.

Raw Leafy Avocado Salad

Ingredients:
2 avocados
1 ½ bunches spinach
½ bunch watercress
1 head Bibb lettuce
1 bunch green onions, green parts only, minced
2 sprigs fresh mint, minced
4 red radishes, minced
juice of 1 lemon
Bragg's Liquid Aminos to taste or wheat-free tamari

Directions:
Scoop avocado into balls with a melon baller.
Clean and chop the greens.
Combine all ingredients and toss with lemon and Bragg's Liquid Aminos or tamari.

Makes 4 servings as a main dish, more as a side.

Raw Lemon Treats

Ingredients:
1 cup chopped, pitted dates
⅓ cup fresh lemon juice
3 tsp freshly grated lemon zest
1 cup raw walnuts
1 cup sesame seeds
½ cup unsweetened dried coconut flakes

Directions:
Place dates, lemon juice and zest, walnuts and sesame seeds in a food processor.
Pulse and blend until completely mixed. The mixture will be slightly sticky.
With dampened hands, roll tablespoons of the mixture into balls.
Roll in coconut and chill until ready to serve.

Makes about 3 dozen TBS-sized balls.

Vegan

Vegan Roasted Butternut Squash Stew

Ingredients:
1 lb dried chickpeas, prepared according to package directions, or 2 large cans
olive oil or coconut oil
2 butternut squashes
2 tsp cardamom powder
2 TBS ground cumin
1 large onion, chopped
6 cloves garlic, minced
2 bunches collard greens, chopped into bite-sized pieces
1 quart vegetable broth
water
salt, pepper, and/or hot sauce to taste

Directions:
Clean and peel the squash and cut into thick rounds, at least an inch thick.
Coat a cookie sheet with olive oil. Lay each round on the sheet and flip it so that there is a film of oil on top.
Roast the squash at 400 degrees for about 25 minutes and flip. Continue roasting until it's fork tender. Allow to cool enough to handle.
Use enough oil to coat the bottom of the soup pot well, sauté cardamom and cumin for a minute, then add the onions and garlic and sauté for about 3 minutes.
Add the collards, chickpeas and vegetable broth and just enough water to cover the greens.
Simmer until the greens are tender enough.
Cut the squash into large chunks and add them to the stew. Heat through and serve.

Serves 8 – 10.

Brussels Sprouts Slaw

Ingredients:
½ cup red onion, sliced very thin
juice of 1 lemon
1 tsp honey
1 tsp Dijon mustard
salt and freshly ground black pepper
2 – 3 TBS olive oil
approx. 3 cups shredded Brussels sprouts

Directions:
Soak the onion slices in a small bowl of cold water for 15 to 20 minutes while you prepare the rest of the ingredients.

Whisk together the lemon juice, honey, mustard and a pinch of salt and pepper. Whisk in 2 TBS of the olive oil until the dressing is emulsified. Taste and see if it wants a little more oil. Set aside.
Trim all of the Brussels sprouts, cutting off yellowed outer leaves and slicing off any hard parts at the root end. Finely shred the sprouts in the food processor.
Put the sprouts in a serving bowl and toss gently with the drained onions and the dressing. Fold in the cheese, taste and adjust seasonings if necessary.

Serves about 4.

Raw Fruit and Nut Ball Variations

The Suppers menu does not provide for much in the way of dessert because we avoid refined foods. Here is one exception: delicious "cookies" made by blending finely chopped dried fruits and nuts. These are extremely sweet, a treat.

Ingredients:
1 ½ cups raisins, rinsed with hot water and drained
1 ½ cups almonds, processed to a fine crumb
1 cup pitted dates
Dried coconut

Directions:
In the food processor, combine the finely processed almonds, raisins and dates. They will start to form a ball.
Take bite-sized pieces of the dough and roll them into a ball, then roll them in coconut or finely chopped nuts.

Makes about 3 dozen.

Variations:
Add 1 TBS cocoa powder to the dough.
Add 1 tsp of cinnamon to the dough.
Add ½ cup dried unsweetened coconut to the dough.
Use other nuts: walnuts, pecans, or filberts.
Use other dried fruit: apricots, figs, currants.
Soak the raisins in the juice of a fresh orange or lemon instead of using hot water.

Vegetarian

Roasted Spaghetti Squash with Olives and Feta
Recipe is taken from Allrecipes.com

Ingredients:
1 spaghetti squash, halved and seeded
2 TBS olive oil
1 onion, chopped
1 ½ cups chopped tomatoes
¾ cup crumbled goat milk feta cheese
3 TBS sliced black olives
2 TBS chopped fresh basil

Directions:
Preheat oven to 350 degrees.
Lightly grease a baking sheet.
Place spaghetti squash cut sides down on the prepared baking sheet, and bake 45 minutes in the preheated oven, or until a sharp knife can be inserted with only a little resistance.
Remove squash from oven, and set aside to cool enough to be easily handled.
Meanwhile, heat oil in a skillet over medium heat.
Sauté onion in oil until tender.
Add garlic and sauté for 2 to 3 minutes.
Stir in the tomatoes, and cook only until tomatoes are warm.
Use a large spoon to scoop the stringy pulp from the squash, and place in a medium bowl.
Toss with the sautéed vegetables, feta cheese, olives, and basil. Serve warm.

Serves 4 – 6.

To get the net carbs that have an influence on your blood sugar, you subtract the fiber from the carbs.

Asparagus Mushroom Soup

Ingredients:
2 yellow onions, chopped
2 bunches asparagus, chopped
1 lb of mushrooms, chopped
preferred fat or olive oil to coat the bottom of the pan
10 cups vegetable stock or water and organic Better than Bouillon
hot pepper sauce to taste

Directions:
Generously coat the bottom of a large pot with olive oil.
Add the onion and stir and cook until a little golden.
Add chopped mushrooms and stock and simmer until mushrooms are soft.
Add asparagus and simmer until just done and still bright green.

Season with hot sauce to taste.

Serves 10 – 12.

Raw Beet Slaw

Ingredients:
1 to 2 medium-sized beets per person, shredded raw
sprinkling of white balsamic vinegar
sprinkling of olive oil
salt, if permitted

Optional: toasted walnuts and crumbled feta cheese

Directions:
Remove tough, rooty bits and scrub the beets.
Shred in a food processor.
Place in a bowl and drizzle on just a bit of vinegar and oil, salt if permitted.
The salad is delicious unadorned, but it holds up with additions of toasted walnuts and/or crumbled feta cheese.

Omnivore

ROYGBIV Salad

Ingredients:
1 red pepper, diced small
3 carrots, shredded
2 oranges, peeled, seeded and diced
1 yellow pepper or one mango, diced small
3 cups greens, like spinach or romaine lettuce
¼ head red cabbage, shredded
6 TBS dried blueberries
1 box black berries, halved if large
½ cup roasted pumpkin seeds
¼ cup toasted sesame seeds

Dressing

Ingredients:
⅔ cup olive oil
juice of 1 lemon
juice of ½ orange
2 TBS light vinegar
1 TBS toasted sesame oil
1 clove garlic
¼ tsp salt
5 drops stevia

Directions:
Combine salad ingredients in a large bowl.
Process dressing ingredients until creamy.
Combine salad and dressing just before serving.

Serves 8 – 10.

Thai Coconut Milk Soup

Ingredients:
extra virgin olive oil or coconut oil to coat bottom of pot
2 leeks, sliced
1 red pepper, slivered
15 large mushrooms, sliced
1 to 2 lbs chicken breast, cut into bite sized chunks
2 cans coconut milk (not lite)
6 cups chicken or vegetable stock
1 block tofu, cubed (optional)

1 large bag or 10 oz. cleaned spinach, chopped
⅓ bunch fresh cilantro, chopped
1 lime, juiced
salt and pepper to taste
hot sauce if desired

Directions:
Coat bottom of soup pot with oil or fat.
Sauté the leeks, red pepper and mushrooms until soft.
Add chicken, coconut milk and stock.
Simmer 15 minutes.
Add tofu, spinach, cilantro, and lime juice and heat until greens are just wilted.
Add salt, pepper and hot sauce to taste.

Serves 8 – 10.

Vegetarians and Omnivores Combined

This is a good model of a recipe that works for a Suppers meeting that combines vegetarians and carnivores as the lentils and lamb are cooked and eaten separately or combined after the cooking is done.

Lentils and Lamb in a Curry Base

Ingredients: Lentils
1 lb package of lentils
1 piece kombu
1 TBS preferred oil or fat (coconut works great)
½ cup tomato sauce
½ cup homemade curry base (see below) or 2 TBS prepared curry paste
salt to taste

Ingredients: Lamb
1 ½ lbs ground lamb
remaining curry base (see below)
1 cup tomato sauce, may need a little water too
salt to taste

Ingredients: Curry Base
oil or preferred fat to coat well the bottom of a large frying pan
2 tsp cardamom
2 TBS coriander powder
3 TBS cumin powder
1 TBS chili powder
2 onions, processed or minced
6 cloves garlic, processed or minced
2 inches of ginger, processed or minced

Directions: Lentils
Rinse and pick through lentils (they often have stones). Add water to cover plus a half inch.
Add kombu, oil, tomato sauce, and curry base or paste.
Simmer until soft, stirring occasionally and adding water if they get too dry.
Remove kombu before serving. Salt to taste.

Directions: Curry Base
Coat the frying pan generously with preferred fat or oil. Heat and add in powder spices and stir constantly for about a minute. They will become fragrant, don't let them get smoky.
Add the onion, ginger, and garlic and cook for three minutes, stirring a few times.
Remove some for the lentils, use the rest for the lamb.

Directions: Lamb
To the remaining curry paste, add the lamb, stir and brown.
Add the tomato sauce and a little water and gently simmer for 20 minutes.

The lentils and lamb may be eaten separately or mixed together.

Red Cabbage and Carrot Salad

Ingredients:
1 lb carrots, shredded
½ head red cabbage, shredded
½ cup figs, chopped (other dried fruit is OK)
1 TBS gomasio or toasted sesame seeds
juice of 1 lemon
juice of 1 orange
2 TBS sesame oil
⅓ cup extra virgin olive oil
salt to taste

Directions:
Mix the carrots, cabbage, sesame seeds, and dried fruit in a salad bowl.
Blend the juices and oils and salt to taste.
Fold in the dressing and serve.

Serves about 8.

Readings

How You Feel is *Data*

Do any of these symptoms sometimes apply to you?

Fatigue
Mental fatigue
Depression
Confusion
Restlessness
Anxiety or panic attacks
Craving
Irritability
Heart palpitations
Excessive sweating
Dizziness
Forgetfulness
Weak spells, hunger, nibbling
Noise and light sensitivity
Nausea
Poor concentration
Moodiness
Insomnia
Mood swings that mimic mental illness

Or perhaps a free floating feeling that something is just not quite right. These symptoms are all at times associated with low blood sugar and the bad mood chemistry that goes along with it. They are gathered from our members and books written by doctors and nutritionists who advocate stabilizing blood sugar as a component of treatment for weight and mood problems, learning issues, and addictions. (See Readings, page 49.) As you can see from the list, the symptoms of low blood sugar are wide-ranging and include physical, mental, emotional, and psychological effects. Many of them are very common complaints, like fatigue, moodiness, and food craving. They are also non-specific, meaning you could experience them for a number of different reasons.

You May Have a Foolish Appetite

If you have these issues *and* you crave processed food, you probably experience "appetite foolishness." Appetite foolishness happens when your body wants food and drinks that destabilize your blood sugar or mood chemistry. The more you eat processed foods to manipulate your mood and energy levels, the more dependent you become on them. The details are complicated, but you don't need to understand them to flip the switch of healing. Briefly, eating carbohydrates raises blood sugar and triggers the release of insulin, the chemical that prevents the sugar levels from going too high. Junk food carbs make this happen a lot faster than healthy carbs like fruits and vegetables. If you've been eating poorly for a long time, you're very likely to experience spikes and crashes, part of the progression toward type 2 diabetes. If you experience comfort or relief from symptoms after eating something sweet, you probably just used sugar as self-medication for low blood sugar and/or the bad mood chemistry that often goes hand in hand.

At Suppers, we consider how you feel *data.* Since one out of three American children are now expected to become diabetic in their lifetimes, we want people to understand the language our bodies use to warn us there's a big problem coming. When it comes to blood sugar, the language is often loud but inarticulate – like anxiety or palpitations – and the feelings can present in different combinations in different people. So one person may be mostly aware of fatigue and poor concentration while another feels hijacked by panic attacks, different problems but both related to how their individual bodies experience poor blood sugar regulation. The good news is that poor blood sugar regulation can usually be improved with diet and lifestyle change. It is a subject that comes up frequently at Suppers meetings, and there is plenty you can do about it.

Sane Person, Crazy Body

Psychologists who include nutrition in their recommendations are typically concerned with the effects of refined foods on focus and mood because they can have such dramatic effects on one's mental and emotional health. (See Ross in Readings, page 49.) They know that the brain is typically the most sensitive organ to poor nutrition. So the spikes and crashes of eating junk food mimic mental health issues. Normalizing blood sugar and mood chemistry with whole food is part of a comprehensive approach to dealing with depression, anxiety, learning issues, obesity, diabetes and problems with alcohol. We call these problems "health relatives" at Suppers because – even though they sound like very different problems – they require similar solutions because they all can be caused by a lifestyle that destabilizes blood sugar and mood chemistry. There are medications that help you manage blood sugar, but there is no medication that cures poor blood sugar regulation and allows you to continue eating however you please. A diet of whole food, stress reduction, and exercise are the way.

First Low Blood Sugar, Then Diabetes

Low blood sugar is *not* the opposite of diabetes (chronically high blood sugar). It is the low range on a roller coaster that many people ride *before they become* type 2 diabetic. In the body's desperate attempts to use insulin to clear toxic levels of sugar out of the blood and store it more safely as fat, the mechanisms break down and for a while, your body overshoots into the low range. You could have bad eating habits and sedentary ways for years before developing type 2 diabetes. During that time your body sends messengers in the form of symptoms like fatigue, food cravings and mood swings. But if you don't understand the language, the symptoms may be misinterpreted as psychological problems, depression, anxiety, mental confusion or even dementia.

Type 3 Diabetes: Alzheimer's Disease

Depending on which research you read, the incidence of Alzheimer's Disease is found 3 or 4 times as often in type 2 diabetics as in the rest of the population. (See Hyman in Readings, page 49.) The scientists are working on sorting out the *nature* of the relationship between blood sugar and Alzheimer's Disease, but the incidence makes one thing clear: there is a lot more Alzheimer's Disease in the diabetic population. Might there be a relationship between the immediate brain affects of poor diet and long term brain effects of poor blood sugar regulation? We don't know. At Suppers, we are not scientists or experts of any kind. We are people who are convinced that by restoring family tables and teaching people how to prepare food from scratch, we can address the *lifestyle* aspects simultaneously of problems rooted in blood sugar regulation and mood chemistry. What we do know is that it makes sense to trust the longest running experiment and return – as much as necessary – to the diet that pre-dates the epidemics.

What Are the Symptoms Trying to Tell Us?

Briefly, the symptoms are telling us our brains are hungry. Brains want to be made mostly of high quality fat, not just any old crappy fat, but fresh fats as they occur in nature. They need to be fed a certain amount of fresh protein, too, enough to provide the building blocks for good mood chemistry. The brain's fuel source is glucose. We get it from eating plant foods. When the glucose supply gets too low for normal brain function, unpleasant symptoms begin, often starting with things like fatigue, mental fatigue or vague feelings that something is not quite right. Experiences differ, but there is a more or less typical progression of events. If you have fatigue or mental fatigue due to poor blood sugar regulation and you don't respond by giving your brain what it's asking for (steady fuel), you'll get more symptoms. The brain's message becomes more urgent, like craving, agitation, and anxiety. These can be the signs that your body is going into an urgent mode to make you get more fuel to the brain. As adrenal stress hormones pump to release stored sugar, you might experience sweats, panic attack, rage, an irrepressible urge to pick up food or drink, or whatever your particular body does when your brain is loudly but inarticulately screaming for nourishment!

Who is Affected?

The people whom we call "health relatives" at Suppers have different health issues, but their solutions are similar because their problems are rooted in the processed food supply. They include people with depression, anxiety, learning issues, obesity, diabetes, and problems with alcohol, and they share similar biochemical and environmental stresses. It is our understanding that their challenges are partly genetic, a combination of how genes, environment, diet, and behaviors interact.

- *People who are physically inactive* are at greater risk. While "exercise" per se may not be required for good health, a life filled with movement is.
- *The poor* are harder hit. Lack of access to good ingredients, recreational opportunities and education make it harder to live well.
- *Specific populations:* The incidence of blood sugar problems is greater in some populations than in others. For example, while it is estimated that one in three American children will end up diabetic, the estimate is one in two for Hispanics, while black Americans are in between. The Native American population is also hard hit with both alcoholism and diabetes. The skyrocketing rates are largely attributable to how poor diet, stress, sedentary lifestyle, social factors, and environmental issues combine with choice and genetic vulnerability.
- *Anyone who is malnourished from processed foods* and other sources of stress is more at risk. They tend to develop appetite foolishness, and they desire to ingest things that temporarily make them feel better but create a bigger problem over time (like drugs do). Malnourishment is self-reinforcing. Once the cycle sets in, cravings can lead to the ingestion of more refined

foods, drinks, and substances that deliver a quick fix of feel-good chemicals and glucose to the brain.

- *People with mental health issues*: Psychiatrists who practice medical nutrition have found blood sugar issues in 30 – 70 percent of psychiatric patients of all diagnostic categories. It's a double whammy for these folks; they are both more likely to crave and eat the exact foods they need to avoid, and they have fewer resources for establishing the kinds of habits that might reduce their suffering. For schizophrenics, the benefits of controlling blood sugar include higher mental function and fewer relapses.
- *Recent newcomers* to the standard American diet are at greater risk. There is research that shows that when people from traditional cultures start eating refined foods and drink, their rate of type 2 diabetes soars. (See Dapice in Readings.)

What Raises Blood Sugar

For the most part, the sugars and starches we eat raise blood sugar. The trick to raising blood sugar without hurting yourself is to not do it too fast. Anything refined or drug-like – like candy, chips, soda, sugar and pizza – raises it so fast that it's a set up for a crash. Alcoholic beverages do too. The ethanol molecule is minute, only 2 ½ times the weight of water. A starch molecule, by comparison, is 250,000 the weight of an alcohol molecule. Both raise blood sugar and alter mood chemistry. But starch can take three or four hours of complicated digestive break down in stomach acids and pancreatic enzymes before its constituents reach the bloodstream. (See Milam and Ketcham in Readings, page 49.) Teeny alcohol zips through membranes. Some is even directly absorbed in the mouth and esophagus. It's an instant band-aid for low blood sugar and foul mood. Eating low starch/high fiber carbohydrates like whole fruit, whole vegetables, and whole grains raises blood sugar appropriately, especially in a balanced diet with protein and high quality fats.

Growth hormones and stress hormones like adrenaline force stored sugar into the blood stream and raise blood sugar. Coffee and cigarettes or anything that stimulates the release of adrenaline ultimately raises blood sugar. Stress raises blood sugar, also because it stimulates the release of adrenaline. Low blood sugar itself causes the raising of blood sugar in two ways. It can send the body into an emergency state that creates cravings for things that will bring the blood sugar levels back into the range for normal brain function. Or it can bring about a stress hormone response that raises blood sugar. It feels extremely unpleasant when this happens. And in a person with poor regulation, whatever makes it rise fast is likely to make it crash.

What is Protective?

* Eating whole foods.
* Exercise, building muscle.
* Lowering stress responses, limiting fight or flight responses.
* Increasing relaxation responses, yoga, meditation, prayer, etc.
* Sleeping and spending enough time in darkness. (See Wiley in Readings, page 49.)
* Drinking enough water.

How Low Blood Sugar Relates to Stress

Nature gave us the ability to pump out chemicals that help us survive in many kinds of stress situations. The adrenal glands make hormones like adrenaline that stimulate us for times of fight or flight. They make cortisol that causes the body to release stored sugar in case the brain levels of sugar go down too low. Stress hormones are *stress* hormones. Regardless of the reason for pumping them – a saber-toothed tiger, a 32-ounce cola, or a bout of low blood sugar – the body experiences stress. Damage takes place whether the stressor is a "real" threat, an imagined threat, or a dietary threat. There are other variables, but stabilizing blood sugar and reducing stress hormones like adrenaline and cortisol can stabilize the vulnerable person in many ways, physically, mentally, and emotionally. We simply can't get control over some sources of stress. But we can reduce *overall* stress by eating stabilizing foods, the kind we teach people to prepare at Suppers.

Correcting the Problem

The answer is simple, but it may not be easy. Because the dietary aspect of poor blood sugar regulation starts with some kind of processed or "de-natured" plant foods, the solution must include returning to unprocessed foods and "re-naturing" the person. Eating whole foods and reducing refined, sweet and starchy ones is the basic formula. Upping the protective factors and reducing the risk factors may require a lot of retraining, cultivating taste buds, and getting support from your family and friends. The Suppers way is to accomplish this in the context of meetings and in the authentic settings of life.

Other Variables

Stabilizing blood sugar is no miracle cure. For those who experience the discomforts listed at the beginning of this document, taking the actions that stabilize blood sugar will resolve the problems *only when the problems are caused by low blood sugar*. Depending on the natural reality of your health challenges, dealing with low blood sugar may be the total but more likely the partial answer. But it is a powerful tool. Eating a diet of whole foods has reduced symptoms and suffering in people with depression, anxiety, learning issues, obesity, diabetes and problems with alcohol. Other diet-related variables in these illnesses are impaired digestion (common in our culture); food sensitivity; environmental allergies as to molds, ethanol, and chemicals; and the need for dietary and supplemental sources of the building blocks of optimal neurotransmitter function. Fortunately, blood sugar stabilization and happy neurotransmitter production require similar diet and lifestyle change because they are closely related. (See Ross in Readings, page 49.)

The Take-home Messages

If you don't remember anything else from this article, remember these few points:

1. How you feel is *data*. Obviously, there's a lot more to good nutrition than just blood sugar regulation. However, blood sugar is one of the most dramatic symptom causers, easy to recognize if you understand your body's language. At Suppers, we work with the assumption that if you live in a way that stabilizes your blood sugar and mood chemistry, then your other diet-related health problems will probably resolve too.

2. Know your numbers: One out of three Americans is headed for type 2 diabetes. How much sense does it make that we can get our blood pressure checked at the mall or the dentist's office but there's a shroud of fear and mystery around checking blood sugar! If your doctor isn't routinely checking, ask to be tested. Plus, a test kit with 10 strips for 10 tests is only $10 at the pharmacy.
3. None of this is rocket science, though scientists can make it sound very complicated when describing the underlying details. If the only message you take away is "Eat real food," it will be enough.
4. You can do this. If you can make a pot of coffee, you can make a pot of soup. The solutions are simple, if not easy. You just need education and support while you find the right diet for your personal needs and develop a palate for real, whole food. That's what we provide at Suppers: enough support to carry you through until junk food loses its appeal and the healthy food becomes delicious. We call it a "logical miracle."
5. Preparing and eating real food is more convenient and less expensive than having depression, anxiety, learning issues, obesity, diabetes, or problems with alcohol, the problems we call "health relatives" at Suppers.

Readings

Beasley, Joseph. (2000). History of Bill W.'s (Co-founder of alcoholics anonymous, A.A.) contribution to nutrition therapy, http://www.addictionend.com/bookonline/section33right04.htm.

Dapice, Ann. (n.d.). Killing us slowly: The relationship between type II diabetes and alcoholism, http://vltakaliseji.tripod.com/Vtlakaliseji/id20.html.

Larson, Joan Mathews. (1997). Seven Weeks to Sobriety.

Hyman, Mark. (2009). The UltraMind Solution.

Milam, James & Ketcham, Katherine. (1983). Under the Influence: A Guide to the Myths and Realities of Alcoholism.

Miller, Merlene & Miller, David. (2005). Staying Clean and Sober: Complementary and Natural Strategies for Healing the Addicted Brain.

National Institute on Alcohol Abuse and Alcoholism. (1996, April). Alcohol and stress. Alcohol Alert, 32, 1 - 5

Pfeiffer, Carl. (1975). Mental and Elemental Nutrients.

Ross, Julia. (2002). The Mood Cure.

Schwarzbein, Diana & Deville, Nancy. (1999). The Schwarzbein Principle.

Wiley, T. S. (2000). Lights Out: Sleep, Sugar, and Survival.

Nutritional Harm Reduction

Many of our Suppers members come to meetings as much for their families as for themselves. Following is a list compiled by members who have succeeded at making incremental changes in their households. Adults and children experienced good to excellent results. Their efforts to practice nutritional harm reduction – gentle, manageable changes over time – have led to:

• reduction of depression	• better moods
• reduction of asthma	• better bowel function
• increased energy	• reduction of ADHD symptoms
• better ability to concentrate	• reduced angry outbursts
• better blood sugar levels	• increased impulse control
• less jitters	• reduction of anxiety, panic

Make Breakfast

The best results we have gotten have happened when people start eating the right breakfast *for them*, as determined by experiments. It usually involves a breakfast combining protein, complex carbohydrates and some high quality fat and NO sweet or artificially sweetened items. Here's why: higher intake of protein and high quality fats can be a therapeutic bridge to better mood chemistry in people who have eaten and drunk too much fuel (carbs) and not enough building blocks (fats and protein) for stable blood sugar and mood chemistry. For others, the experiments reveal that a vegan approach brings them the greatest energy. You can find out which type you are by trying our breakfast challenge and getting real data about your body:
http://www.thesuppersprograms.org/Documents/Activities/BreakfastChallenge_Jan10.pdf

Teach Them the Difference Between a Snack and Dessert

Snacks are the same food you would eat at a meal; they help children grow. They have nutritional value. They're healthy for adults too. Snacks include leftovers, fruits, vegetables, nuts, seeds, etc. Desserts are everything else: they should only be eaten on a belly full of real food (high fiber vegetables and fruits, good fats, and lean protein). That means you don't have to totally vilify chips, candy, cookies, bagels, soft drinks, and other junk, which would cause rebellion. They just have to start looking like dessert instead of a snack. People who experience fatigue or mood swings after eating wheat, dairy, sugar or any food that causes an unwanted reaction may need to avoid these items entirely. Cravings are also a tip-off that your body doesn't tolerate a food.

Replace Favorite Foods with Healthier Versions

Keep the family in the discussion. Start with small changes like replacing big-name junk food items containing hydrogenated fats and high fructose corn syrup with the health food store varieties. Here's why: although they still contain too much blood sugar destabilizing processed ingredients, they eliminate the worst food poisons and are a step in the right direction. Our members have braved the objections and been happy to realize that as favorite junk foods are less available, healthier versions of junk food gain acceptance.

Introduce Water as a Beverage Option

Keep a fresh pitcher in the fridge. Put the pitcher on the table at snacks and meals. At the same time, reduce purchases of sugared or artificially sweetened soft drinks. Expect sabotage and/or rebellion; that's fine.

Beat Them to It

Have fresh fruit, cut up veggies, nuts, seeds, hummus, cheese (if they tolerate it) and leftovers ready when they are hungry. Let the salad or a plate of fruits and veggies be the first thing on the table while you prepare the rest of the meal. If no adult is there and they are regularly feeding themselves, this is part of the problem. This is not to make anybody feel guilty; it's just to acknowledge that without an adult taking charge, most kids will gravitate to the drug-like food. The same goes for adults. Distinguish a treat from a trigger. If a food causes cravings and unwanted eating, it's a trigger. It's easier to not keep it in the house.

Buy Mostly Food That Has No Label

The trouble starts when there is a list of ingredients. The food that will turn your health around doesn't need a label because it contains only one, readily obvious thing: one chicken, two apples, three yams, etc. Of particular concern are flavor enhancers like MSG and artificial sweeteners, which are particularly toxic to brain cells when blood sugar is low.
http://www.thesuppersprograms.org/Documents/Information/FoodAdditives.pdf

Exercise Control at the Grocery Store and You Won't Have to at Home

The most important time to exercise control is before junk comes into the house. If you buy it and try to control it at home, it's a lot harder. One couple started using the babysitting service at the grocery store so they could take the time to read labels and make selections without the children's input. In general, the whole food is in the periphery of the store, and the junk is in the aisles. Avoid aisles.

Take Them Out for the Treats

Head in the direction of letting the home pantry contain only healthy foods. Set a clear boundary. Let a trip to the ice cream store or bakery (if they tolerate some dairy, wheat and sugar) be a real treat because it doesn't take place every day. If something takes place every day, it's not a treat; it's the expected norm. If the treat triggers mood change, whining, or unwanted eating, it wasn't a treat, it was a trigger.

Pay Attention to Digestion

How you digest is data. Bloating, diarrhea, constipation, excessive farting, foul smelling gas, and belching are all indications that a body is not digesting well. Good digestion is important because you are NOT what you eat. You are only what you absorb of what you eat. If digestive problems don't clear up with an improved diet, a consultation with a nutritionist may be in order.

Do Not Ask Your Kids or Yourself "Does It Taste Good?"

Nutritional harm reduction facilitates transition. If it were easy to switch from our favorite junk foods to a diet of whole foods, we would have done it by now. Here's a promise: As you eat healthier, whole foods, your body will transition from "Yuck" and disappointment to acceptance to enjoyment. This is a leap of faith. In Suppers terms, once the brain makes the association between whole foods and better mood chemistry, tastes develop for the healthy foods. It took one of our members a few months to develop a taste for vegetables, most others started feeling the effects and desiring more salads immediately. Members who were not getting enough protein felt less anxious and depressed as soon as they started eating enough to meet their individual needs. This is very positive reinforcement.

Talk to Them

Let spouses, friends, and children know how important it is to make these changes and why. This is not a democracy. *Parents* determine the boundaries about what comes into the house. Friends don't get a vote in what you eat.

Learn Which Jobs are Yours and Which Belong to the Kids

When it comes to feeding and eating, the division of labor can get pretty confusing. Here are the recommendations for people who need to stabilize blood sugar and mood chemistry:

The Parents' job is to:

1. Bring into the house only the healthy foods you want the family to eat.
2. Exclude foods that act like bargaining chips (you know they are more drug-like if people lobby to get them).
3. Model the eating behavior you want from your children.
4. Provide meals and appropriate snacks. If you aren't home to monitor controversial items, it's easier for everybody if you do not keep them in the house.
5. Include the family in as many steps as possible: eating together at a table, preparing the food, picking the food, even growing the food.
6. Avoid hovering, micromanaging, prodding, bargaining. None of these is necessary if you have only healthy whole food – and no triggers – in the house.
7. Observe how they react/respond to foods and drinks. Take charge of food elimination and challenge experiments if a dietary culprit is suspected.
8. Don't worry yet about a "balanced diet." Balance comes *after* they acquire the taste for whole food.
9. Observe responses to decide what's a treat and what's a trigger. Treats are favorite foods that do not lead to unwanted eating and behavior. Triggers lead to unwanted eating or behaviors.

The Child's job is to:

1. Decide what they want to eat from the healthy foods available.
2. Decide how much to eat.
3. Participate in as many steps as possible: eating together at a table, preparing the food, picking the food, even growing the food.

Expect Sabotage and/or Rebellion

These changes are not going to be greeted favorably by anyone who is stuck on junk food's hook. Once you have determined what the boundaries will be, parents are the keepers of the family health. Resistance, hostility, rebellion and spousal or friend sabotage are normal points on the trajectory of change.

Schedule a Clean-Out-the-Pantry Day

This is a family event. Once you have started making changes and the family is accepting some healthier alternatives, make a project of reading all the labels in the pantry and throwing out whatever does not meet the new family standard. One mom gave her kids two choices: keeping all their favorite breads, salad dressings, and canned soup and never having dessert OR switching to the healthier versions of staples and enjoying (health food store) desserts. The kids got on board in spite of the obvious manipulation.

Cook With Each Others' Kids

They often handle the information better if it comes from somebody other than Mom or Dad. Two moms in our group asked their sons to give them the present of attending Suppers for Teens as their Christmas or birthday present to Mom. The boys had control over the ingredients in the pots of soup and stew they took home. Pride in the process, greater interest in cooking, and curiosity about the food channel followed.

Observe Reactions

Everybody reacts differently to foods. There is no sense being a control freak about sugar if gluten grains are the big problem. It can get complicated to sort out food sensitivities, but here is a good rule of thumb: The more wedded someone is to a particular food or drink, the more likely it is to be acting like a drug *in that individual.* Treating oneself to a bit of chocolate if one feels like an addict around chocolate is like giving a recovering alcoholic the reward of just one drink. Whining, craving, and lobbying for specific foods are clear signs that it's time to check for food sensitivities.

70 – 85% of the Whole Food Ideal is a Good Goal

70 – 85% of what's ideal for you is a good goal *except* for foods that are triggers or like drugs *for you,* the items from which you must abstain. That leaves plenty of room for treats as long as they don't trigger undesired eating or brain symptoms.

The Clear Solution: Return – as Much as Possible – to the Behaviors that Predate these Epidemics.

Diet and lifestyle changes can help you delay, reverse, and even heal the problem. The way in to the problem suggests the way out: If eating and drinking processed foods and beverages got you into this mess to begin with, then changing to whole foods is the way out. At the very least, you can mitigate the damage by thoughtfully addressing the content, timing, digestion, and circumstances under which you eat food. We know that returning to the foods and behaviors that predate the epidemics is safe; for everything else we are lab rats.

Conclusion

Our number one national addiction is not alcohol, drugs or cigarettes. It's food. Poor quality food is responsible for more preventable health and mental health problems than any other source. And the national menu of processed foods is so drug-like that many of us have lost the ability to enjoy the taste of real food, food that supports life. This makes the standard American diet a gateway to obesity and diabetes, addictions, and many mental health problems including anxiety, depression, and learning issues. We cannot abstain from eating. That leaves us with nutritional harm reduction.

To determine if you or someone you know is a good candidate for a Suppers Programs, ask yourself the following question: Do I believe that the food I eat has a significant influence on my health, cravings, mood, behavior, and/or mental function? If yes, it is time to examine how much of a role is played by food. The early signs of being in the process that is leading one out of three American children to a diagnosis of diabetes are often weight gain and brain symptoms: depression, anxiety, poor behavior, and learning issues. This is because the brain is very vulnerable to poor nutrition.

Preparing for Change/Setting Good Goals

In order to practice nutritional harm reduction, it's going to require changing some habits. When changing a behavior, particularly one that involves a drug or drug-like food, you'll need good goals and lots of support.

Good goals – no matter what they are – share certain things in common. They are clear and doable. They are specific and concrete. They are realistic. And they require you to focus on what *you* can change. Of course, at Suppers, you can rely on the support of therapeutic friends.

Although we state goals in the positive, there is often a negative motivation. What needs to change? How important is it to fix this? What are the consequences of not doing so? Whatever you want to accomplish, you can break it down into manageable goals. You've come to Suppers, you had some likely outcome in mind.

Some goals aren't enjoyable. So a good question to ask yourself might be: How important is it that I accomplish this (rather than do I feel like doing it)? If working on a goal is enjoyable but not important, it may still be a good beginner goal if you need to experience early success. So, for example, a good beginner goal is something you already do and give yourself credit for: I will attend a weekly Suppers meeting.

If it's not enjoyable, but it's important, you might get some fuel from answering the question "How is what I am currently doing working out for me?"

Examples

A good goal is really clear.
I will go to bed at 10 p.m., NOT
I wish I had more energy.

Focus on what you can do, not what you can get somebody else to do.
I will do a crossword puzzle in the check out line, NOT
I will complain to the manager for displaying all that candy at the check out.

Focus on healthy solutions.
I will eat two fruits per day, NOT
I will skip meals to save on calories.

Be specific.
I will eat an apple daily, NOT
I will eat more fruit.

Make it measurable.
I will prepare one Suppers meal per week for my family, NOT
I will cook more frequently.

Make it realistic for you.
I will walk ½ hour per day, four times per week, NOT
I will exercise two hours every day.

Make it affordable now.
I will walk with Betty three times a week for an hour, NOT
I will start saving for that fabulous in-home gym.

Make it concrete.
I will use 50% of my grocery budget for single, fresh, whole food, NOT
I will buy healthy food.

Keep the focus positive.
I will eat my favorite sweets exclusively as dessert after a meal of whole food, NOT
I will avoid sweets all day until after dinner.

Make it an outcome you can succeed at by doing the behavior.
I will eliminate sugar from my diet, NOT
I will lose 10 pounds this month.

Sample Questionnaire: Preparing for Change
A sample has been prepared for you; see answers in *italics*.

Read an example of how to prepare for change. You could do this alone, but it might work better doing it with a therapeutic friend.

I am thinking about making the following change: *Quitting caffeine.*

1. Name the reason you think something must change.
I can't stand the anxiety anymore.

2. Name benefits of staying the same.
I love coffee, it starts my day.

3. Name benefits of changing.
The lift is short lived. I feel addicted to caffeine and think I will feel more stable if I quit.

4.   Describe the difference you want to experience.
I will feel less panicky.

5. Name a small change one could make that would lead to the desired outcome.
Reducing the intake.

6. Acknowledge how you feel when thinking about making the change.
Mixed, scared, might fail.

7. How important is it? You can use a scale of 1 to 10.
I think it's about 8. I hate how I feel.

8. What makes it so important?
It's affecting how I relate to my family. My head spins more and more as I lose tolerance for caffeine.

9. What else will have to happen to make change possible?
I will need my family to be supportive. I have to stop eating doughnuts because I can't have one without the other.

10. What might sabotage the process?
If I meet friends as usual at the diner Saturday mornings.

11. How will you handle the potential sabotage?
I have to have some honest conversations with them before I do this.

12. What will happen if you stayed the same?
I will continue to feel addicted, spinning, a slave to caffeine.

13. How can the change be broken down into small, manageable pieces?
I can talk to my family before changing anything.
I can tell my friends this is coming and to not expect me for breakfast until I accomplish this.
I can eat protein at breakfast to help stabilize me.
I can take supplements to help prevent the headaches I would usually get.
I can do it in stages rather than cold turkey.

14. What support would help you accomplish this?
If my family knew I was going to be a bear for a week, they could not take it personally when I am cranky and nasty. I need to ask for their support.

15. Who can provide that support?
Kids and husband. Come to think of it, I should tell my boss too.

16. How will you know when you have achieved the change?
I will be off coffee for as long as it takes to resist the urge to have it without feeling sorry for myself.

Preparing for Change

Now try your hand at writing down a goal that is concrete, measurable, and doable; something you can accomplish yourself or with a willing supporter, not something that requires recruiting some one else.

I am preparing to make the following change:

1. Name the reason you think something must change.

2. Name benefits of staying the same.

3. Name benefits of changing.

4. Describe the difference you want to experience.

5. Name a small change one could make that would lead to the desired outcome.

6. Acknowledge how you feel when thinking about making the change.

7. How important is it? You can use a scale of 1 to 10.

8. What makes it so important?

9. What else will have to happen to make change possible?

10. What might sabotage the process?

11. How will you handle the potential sabotage?

12. What will happen if you stayed the same?

13. How can the change be broken down into small, manageable pieces?

14. What support would help you accomplish this?

15. Who can provide that support?

16. How will you know when you have achieved the change?

When you're ready to commit to a new behavior, write your plan for the week and check it off each time you accomplish what you set out to do.

Plan for the Week

Example
I will _____walk_____ (Do what?)
_____2 blocks_____ (How much?)
_____before breakfast_____ (When?)

Monday
I will _____ (Do what?)
_____ (How much?)
_____ (When?)

Tuesday
I will _____ (Do what?)
_____ (How much?)
_____ (When?)

Wednesday
I will _____ (Do what?)
_____ (How much?)
_____ (When?)

Thursday
I will _____ (Do what?)
_____ (How much?)
_____ (When?)

Friday
I will _____ (Do what?)
_____ (How much?)
_____ (When?)

Saturday
I will _____ (Do what?)
_____ (How much?)
_____ (When?)

Sunday
I will _____ (Do what?)
_____ (How much?)
_____ (When?)

60

Things to Try

Beginner Questionnaire

Do your health challenges relate to the food you're eating? Suppers can help anyone with diet- and lifestyle-related health and mental health challenges, and we're especially useful for people with issues related to blood sugar and mood chemistry. Take our Beginner Questionnaire to see if Suppers is right for you.

1. Does at least one of the following problems occur in your biological family?
    ___ Obesity or struggles with weight
    ___ Diabetes or hypoglycemia
    ___ Alcoholism or problem drinking

2. Does at least one of the following problems occur in your biological family?
    ___ Depression
    ___ Anxiety
    ___ Learning issues
    ___ Insomnia or inadequate sleep

3. Do you personally experience at least one item from both questions 1 and 2?

4. Can you take or leave coffee? chocolate? pastries? chips? cookies? bread? soft drinks? alcoholic beverages?

5. For women: Do or did your answers to question 4 depend on the time of the month?

6. Do you skip breakfast?

7. Is your evening weight more than two pounds greater than your morning weight?

8. Do you mostly eat meals made from whole foods (like fresh vegetables, meat or fish, legumes and whole grains)?

9. Are you satisfied with how you manage your stress level?

10. Do you regularly engage in exercise or some meaningful physical activity?

11. Do you eat regularly at the family table?

12. Do you have satisfying connections with other people?

Interpretation

Questions 1 – 3
If you answered yes to all three, you are a good candidate for Suppers. Your answers suggest that the solutions to your health challenges need to include diet and lifestyle style change to support stable blood sugar and mood chemistry.

Question 4
If you feel pulled in by these items, you may have a relationship with addictive items in the food supply that are jeopardizing your health or sobriety and affecting mood, sleep, and mental function. Again, we'd like to invite you to try Suppers, or Suppers for Sobriety if you're in recovery. Over time, we can give you the support you need to reduce your dependence on drug-like foods and beverages and develop a taste for foods that promote health.

Question 5
Increased cravings and mood swings around the cycle can sometimes be normalized with a stabilizing diet. At very least, stabilizing includes a healthy diet.

Question 6
Some of the most dramatic improvements we have seen have been around breakfasting behavior: relief from panic attacks, relief from depression, relief from cravings. At Suppers you'll learn why and get support finding what works for your body.

Question 7
If your evening weight is more than two pounds greater than your morning weight, it is likely to be an indication that your body does not tolerate something you are eating or drinking. True weight does not go up in a day. Fluid retention, or edema, can come from consuming something toxic or something to which you are allergic or "hypersensitive." The culprits are likely to be things that are "comfort" foods, i.e., things that give you a temporary lift but set you up for a crash later.

Question 8
All of the health issues listed in questions 1 and 2 relate to food and beverage processing and the havoc it wreaks on blood sugar and mood chemistry. If these items were not in the food supply, the problems would hardly exist. If you would like to learn how to prepare whole foods, we hope you will join us for Suppers.

Question 9
Stress itself is very destabilizing for blood sugar and mood chemistry and can itself increase the chances of relapse. At Suppers you will learn very simple techniques to reduce stress and become more aware of the effects of foods and stress on your body. If you experience a combination of the challenges in questions 1 and 2, your diet itself may be a source of stress. At Suppers, the #1 way we can help is by supporting you as you find the best way for you to eat. A close second is learning to manage stress better, through breathing exercises, the camaraderie of Suppers tables, guided meditations, and body awareness exercises.

Question 10
Everybody already knows we need exercise and meaningful physical activity. The habit is hard to establish. Your therapeutic friends at Suppers meetings can help you set doable goals, even walk or exercise together with you.

Question 11
Research on the positive effects of eating at a family table is clear: Children who eat regular meals with their parents are at reduced risk for alcohol, tobacco and drug use. If you don't know how to make family tables a reality in your household, we hope you'll accept our invitation to Suppers.

Question 12
Good human connections are healing; they reduce stress and provide a healthier source of pleasure. At Suppers you will find people who actively practice nonjudgment as part of our commitment to healing for the greatest number.

Breakfast Challenge

How will I know if food is causing my problems with mood and energy? Find out at breakfast time, when you get the best possible read on how your body relates to foods.

Try the Suppers Breakfast Challenge

If you have any combination of:

* Strong preference for refined carbs: candy, cake, chips, soda, and white bread
* Irregular breakfast habits or habits of sweet or starchy breakfast
* Unsatisfactory energy levels

AND

Depression	Obesity
Anxiety	Diabetes
Learning Issues	Problems with alcohol
Confirmed or Suspected Eating Disorder	

Then the Suppers breakfast challenge will give you important *data* about your body. All you need to do is try four different breakfasts and note how you feel.

Days 1 and 2 Do what you usually do
Days 3 and 4 Have scrambled eggs with some green vegetables and NOTHING ELSE
Days 5 and 6 Have unsweetened oatmeal or whole grain cereal and milk or milk substitute and NOTHING ELSE
Days 7 and 8 Have breakfast chili and NOTHING ELSE

If you would like to try a vegan raw fruit option, substitute a fruit smoothie (recipe below) for the eggs or chili.

Rationale: If you have a combination of the issues that The Suppers Programs deal with – depression, anxiety, learning issues, obesity, diabetes and/or problems with alcohol – AND a strong preference for refined carbohydrates, it's *data*. Our members usually start improving when they find the right kind of breakfast *for them*. For some, oatmeal works. For most, a meal that combines adequate protein, high quality fat, and low starch vegetables brings a big boost of energy, holds off cravings, and levels out moods. And for some of our members, a strict vegan approach emphasizing in-season fruits has brought vibrant health. But you won't know which works best for you until you try an experiment and observe the results.

Just note how you feel through the day. If you must have coffee, wait until an hour after you eat, or you'll sabotage the experiment. If you can't wait for your coffee, that's *data*.

Breakfast Chili: A super easy way to make a big batch

* Place enough olive oil in a soup pot to coat the bottom.
* On medium heat, brown 2 lbs of ground turkey.

- Add 4 cups of high fiber vegetable, like finely shredded cabbage.
- Add 2 cans of drained kidney, black, or preferred beans.
- Add 1 small jar of salsa and 1 small jar of tomato sauce after reading the labels to make sure there is no form of sugar or corn syrup in them.
- Depending on the amount of liquid in the salsa, you will need to add some water.
- Add 1 TBS of chili powder, or to taste.
- Add salt to taste, if it is not restricted for you.
- Optional: up to 6 cups of chopped vegetables, like peppers, onion, carrots, greens

Let it simmer until the water steams off and it is the consistency you like, about ½ hour.

In the ideal world, your ingredients would be organic and fresh. This is not the ideal world.

Follow the Suppers principle of nutritional harm reduction
http://www.thesuppersprograms.org/Documents/Information/NutritionalHarmReduction_Tips.pdf
and use the highest quality ingredients you can *without stressing over it.*

Vegetarians

Although most of our members do better with some animal protein, we also see great success among vegetarians. Vegans can try the challenge with black bean chili. Those who eat eggs but not meat can add an egg to the menu. The goal is to feel the effects on your body of various foods. Those who wish to try a fruity vegan approach can make smoothies by processing 2 – 4 TBS full fat coconut milk with fruits like: 1 banana, ½ cup mixed berries, 1 peach, 1 pineapple wedge and some greens, such as a few leaves of kale.

Tracking

Choose a few things you'd like to track like energy, mood, alertness, concentration, number of hours before hunger sets in, cravings. Make note of how you feel throughout the day.

	Breakfast	Morning	Midday	Afternoon	Evening
Day 1	Oats and OJ	hungry, fuzzy brain	hoagie, tired	ready for a drink	cranky
Day 2					
Day 3					
Day 4					
Day 5					
Day 6					
Day 7					
Day 8					

Sample Guided Relaxation

To quiet ourselves and help us relax, slow down and digest our food, some one who can pace him/herself to a slow rhythm can read this short relaxation exercise.

Take a breath… and release.

If you care to, close your eyes and just notice how it feels to be in your body.

Let your feet rest flat on the floor. Place your hands in your lap. And sit comfortably erect.

Take a breath… and release.

Notice where your body makes contact with the outside world…

The feel of your feet in your shoes…

The pressure of your buttocks against the seat...

The pressure of your back against the back of the chair…

And now the feel of air as it enters your lungs…

Notice what your tongue can feel inside your mouth…

Now bring your awareness to the tip of your nose and just notice what it feels like when the air moves into your nostrils when you breathe in…

And then how it feels as you breathe out…

Scan your body for areas of tightness or tension…

And when you find one, breathe into it…

And release.

Now bring your awareness back to the room and when you're ready, please open your eyes.

Play it to the End (Story with Exercise to Try)

This idea is not original, but I got a lot of credit at our meeting for bringing this idea into our group. It's an activity called "Play it to the End."

The issue on the table was self-sabotage. Everybody in our group attends Suppers in the hope of turning around some long-term eating patterns that have gotten us into a lot of trouble. Some of us are literally digging our graves with our forks. We've eaten out of control until the diagnosis of diabetes stirs the fear of God in us. Our eyes were wide open. Every time we put something in our mouths, we were there (if not actually present). We knew it ran in our families. Still, we dug deeper.

One of our number said her best form of self-sabotage was continuing to socialize with people whose favorite activities were eating and drinking. Another said she could trick herself every time by telling herself, "Oh I'll just eat two." Wrong. Two equals twenty. We all had experience with the skip-breakfast-save-calories logic. Bad. But the form of self-sabotage we all did over and over was seducing ourselves into eating with blind anticipation and good memories of pleasurable eating that never, however, played out to remembering the consequences too. However many times I anticipated with relish some tasty treat, that's how many times my memory tricked me.

So my contribution to Suppers is the activity called "Play It To The End." Here's how it works.

The speaker recounts a made-up story in which he or she indulges in a favorite but problematical food, but they have to tell the whole story including the part about the consequences, "playing the tape to the end." Here's mine:

"We are at a reception and the dessert table is beckoning. There is a cheesecake dripping with cherry sauce, three kinds of chocolate cake, a key lime pie, champagne flutes of chocolate mousse and five kinds of cookies. I take slivers of each of the chocolate cakes. I am in heaven. The one with a layer of chocolate ganache is stunningly delicious. I go back for a big slice, a wedge of key lime pie and a few cookies. For 10 minutes, I'm in bliss. I swallow the last bite. It's all in my stomach. I think about the calories, the fact that it's 9:00 p.m. and how I'll probably be up for three hours in the middle of the night after so much sugar and stimulation. I sleep lousy. I feel bloated and disgusting. I kick myself for forgetting the consequences of late night blasts of sugar."

I have imagined partial scenarios just like this over and over but for some reason remembering the whole experience doesn't come automatically. The automatic part of my brain only recalls the anticipation and eating. It requires my full conscious participation to recall the consequences. I have spared myself many nights of lost sleep since I learned to play my eating scenarios to the end.

Exercise: Let members who care to share completing the imaginary experience of anticipating, eating and feeling the consequences of eating a food that acts more like a drug for them. To help you get started, you may use a prompt:

There was a bowl of chocolates on the table…
Everybody wanted to go for ice cream…
I am passing my favorite fast food joint and…

Directions for Setting Up a Food/Mood Observation Notebook

If you find it difficult to observe how you feel, your therapeutic friends at Suppers meetings will help you begin. You can ask for help: phone calls, e-mails, food prep, shared meals between meetings. Skeptical and even well intentioned family and friends can sabotage the process. Get help.

Step 1: Get a notebook.

Step 2: Make a statement about what you hope to get from food journaling, something like: I will identify which foods anchor me and which foods destabilize me.

Step 3: Select your "flag words," words that remind you what you want to keep track of. They might include: fatigue, hunger, cravings, mental clarity, mood, number of hours of sleep, productivity, sense of well being, thought patterns, arguments, jitters, bloating, nausea.

Step 4: Journal daily as follows:

- Note morning and evening weight. If it is more than a couple pounds different, it is a good bet that you are holding water in response to something you are eating or drinking. If weighing yourself is way too triggering, it's OK, go to the next direction.

- On the left side of each page, write the date, time of day, and what you ingest for 24 hours. Write everything and don't change a thing just because you are taking notes. No one is watching. Let the only criterion for success be accuracy.

- On the right side, list observations using your flag words as reminders.

Patterns may emerge, like you always get sleepy in the late morning when you have a bagel and OJ for breakfast or you get congested when you have peanut butter & jelly and milk for lunch. If you suspect a food is trouble for you, you can test it by doing an elimination test.

Step 5: Elimination test:

When you think you know what may be causing your problems, you can test it. This is actually more accurate than some medical tests, but it does take some work and support. It's simple, but maybe not easy.

To test a suspected food:

- Eliminate it from your diet 100% for four to 14 days (experts disagree on the time, longer is probably more accurate). It has to be 100% or the test doesn't work. Grill waiters, read all labels, get a therapeutic friend to help you prepare single, whole, fresh ingredients. Ask for support, the offending foods are often the ones you think you can't live without because you have a drug-like relationship with them.

- Take your notes several times daily.

- After at least four days, test it by having a good portion of it and note how you feel for the next two days (yes, some foods take over a day to create the symptom).

- Take notes on how you feel when you re-introduce the suspected item.

If re-introduced foods produce symptoms, it's *data.*

If you do react, wait two days on the pure diet before testing another food.

The best results are likely to come if you eliminate all processed foods and highly allergenic foods before the challenge. This is because people who are intolerant of one food are likely to be intolerant of many. Remember the big culprits are gluten grains (wheat, rye, barley), dairy, sugar, and runners up: soy, corn, chocolate and coffee. Of course, alcohol can do it too.

If you can face going off wheat but not dairy for a couple weeks, stick with the spirit of nutritional harm reduction and test wheat. There are very few times at Suppers when you have to be rigid, and elimination testing is one of the few. To clear the items from your system and accurately test, your body needs the total break (4 – 14 days) for you to experience how liberating it feels to be off a food that is affecting your brain, mood, behavior, energy level, etc.

Remember: The only criterion for success is your ability to make accurate observations. At Suppers, there's no judgment, *just data!*

Sample Food/Mood Observation Chart

Select key tracking words so you remember what to observe.

These might include:
alertness, anxiety, depression, concentration, sleep, memory, cravings, energy, mood, productivity

Example:

Time of Day	Ate/Drank	Observations
Morning		
8:00	coffee, dry bagel	
10:30		sleepy, fuzzy head
10:45	coffee, chocolate bar	feel better
noon		really hungry
12:15	big salad	not satisfied, moody
Afternoon		
2:00	coffee	hard to focus
		feel unproductive
4:00		thinking about a drink
5:15		foul mood, irritated
		hard to stay alert driving home
Evening		
6:00	two drinks	relief
	salty nuts	
7:15	steak, salad, potatoes	energy low, feel OK
10:30	big glass of water	exhausted
		slept pretty well

Food/Mood Observation Chart

Select key tracking words so you remember what to observe.

Time of Day	Ate/Drank	Observations
Morning		
Afternoon		
Evening		

Sample Personal Progress Observation to Share at Meetings (Inventory)

If you wish to have periodic meetings at which you monitor and share your progress, here is a suggested format for organizing your thoughts. Choose your own criteria and be sure to leave out the ones you don't want to track (for example, some of us are better off not focusing on weight). Jot brief notes or rate 1 to 10. You can set up your own chart of things to track. A sample follows.

Date

Habits and Behaviors
> hours of sleep
> breakfast habits
> exercise
> cooking
> getting quiet time
> eating new foods
> household changes
> family eating habits

Feelings
> hours until hungry after breakfast
> mood
> enjoyment of veggies
> enjoyment of fruit
> interest in junk
> pleasure in cooking
> energy/mental energy
> stress
> sense of empowerment
> sense of feeling toxic

Body
> weight (or how clothes fit)
> weight difference, a.m./p.m.
> allergies
> meds
> joints
> skin
> congestion, postnasal drip
> bowel function
> cravings
> blood sugar or A 1 C
> other tests

Own Comments

Changes Contemplating

Experiments to try

Kernels

Blood Sugar/Mood Chemistry Roller Coaster Chart of Feelings

The starting assumption at Suppers is that if we each ate the way we need to eat to have stable blood sugar and mood chemistry, we'd be eating the right way for us. The mechanisms of blood sugar and mood chemistry are complicated in the details, but easy to understand in practical terms. Our experience of these physical events is feelings and sensations. If you have a "relationship" with refined carbohydrates (soda, chips, candy, cake, pasta, bread or alcohol) and you experience these feelings, it may be important data.

Below you will find a description of how people can feel when their blood sugar ranges high, normal, low or very low. Nobody experiences all of these feelings; it's a matter of biological individuality which ones you do experience. But they are giving you important feedback about what's going on in your body because how you feel is *data!*

High Blood Sugar: Diabetic Range
Pre-diabetic (visiting highs but not staying high) or T-2 diabetic (chronically high) you may feel:
>OK
>Fatigued
>Sluggish

Normal Blood Sugar: The Range for Normal Brain Function
You may feel:
>Clear
>Calm
>No thoughts of food or stimulants

Low Blood Sugar: Hypoglycemic Range
You may feel many different kinds of brain symptoms and uncomfortable feelings:

Mental/Learning	Mood	Behavior	Physical
Poor concentration	Depressed	Laziness	"Spent"
Confusion	Anxious	Act on cravings	Cravings
Mental fatigue	Dissatisfied	Act on impulses	Plunging
ADD or ADHD	Cranky	Aggressive	Jittery

Very Low/Adrenal Stress Hormone Response
You may feel:

Desperate thoughts	Panic	Rage trigger	Palpitations
Survival mode	Anger/rage	Disordered eating	Sweating
No learning	Extreme swings	Binging trigger	Shaking

Coma
The very uncomfortable feelings of low and very low sugar indicate how much your body does NOT want to let you go into a coma. They are *data!*

Dietary Guidelines for Stability

These ideas were drawn from doctors, nutritionists, and nutrition-oriented psychologists who use diet and supplements to stabilize blood sugar and provide the building blocks for neurotransmitters. Suppers does not make specific recommendations on nutrients. They may be crucial for stability in certain individuals, particularly certain biological types of alcoholics. For more information, please see the resource section for readings (page 49), especially The Mood Cure (Ross), The Crazy Makers (Simontacchi), Dr. Bernstein's Diabetes Solution and The Diabetes Diet (Bernstein), and Seven Weeks to Sobriety (Larson).

1. Eat mostly whole, single, fresh foods.

2. Avoid refined foods: flour, sugar, soft drinks, even sugar substitutes and processed foods. Frozen is better than canned.

3. Get them as fresh as you can, like locally grown produce in season.

4. Drink water: half your weight in ounces is a good guideline if you are detoxifying.

5. Do not let yourself get so hungry you start craving. Have a small meal or nourishing snack BEFORE the symptoms of low blood sugar set in. You'll come to find you have a pattern and you can use food strategically.

6. Snacks are the exact same food you would eat for meals. None of them come prepared in packages. Choose whole fruits, nuts, a small portion of protein (meat, eggs, fish, fowl, beans, seeds and nuts). Some people can tolerate dairy foods, others must avoid it. The Suppers menu avoids milk products so members can learn how to eat to correct digestive problems and reduce cravings.*

7. Limit the grain-based foods you eat and choose only whole grains, like brown rice. Some people can handle bread and wheat products. Others must avoid it. The Suppers menu avoids gluten grains like wheat so members can learn how to eat to correct digestive problems and reduce cravings.*

* Wheat products and milk may cause trouble in recovering people and people with health problems that include blood sugar regulation and digestive problems. In general, if eating these foods elevates mood or makes you feel gleeful and/or you have problems with constipation, diarrhea, reflux, flatulence, or "brain fog," a test period without dairy and wheat products is worth a try. Suppers recipes don't include wheat or dairy because they can slow down the recovery process in certain people. Once the gut heals, they may be OK again.

8. Eat foods in combination, getting a balance of high quality fats (like olive oil), high quality protein, high fiber fresh vegetables and fruits. There will be fewer problems with insulin insensitivity and low blood sugar if you "oppose" carbohydrates (sugars and starches) by eating them with other foods. For example, if you decide to eat a piece of pie, do it only after a complete meal. It will do less damage in terms of blood sugar than having it on an empty stomach.

9. Sit down regularly at a table to home cooked meals with people who care about you and no TV, noise, harsh lighting, or other interference.

10. Choose:

    - *Protein:* All meats, fish, fowl, seeds, nuts, legumes (beans) and if you can handle it, dairy. If milk products make you really happy or crave or make you constipated or produce mucous symptoms, hold off for a period of months.

    - *Fruits and Vegetables:* Eat anything fresh and whole. If you don't have a taste for vegetables, start slowly adding it in a little at a time. Be sure to eat some raw foods each day to restore enzymes (protein structures produced by living organisms that make body processes happen).

    - *Fats and oils:* Freshness is critical. Most vegetable oils are fragile and become rancid on the shelf. Reasonable quantities of extra virgin olive oil are beneficial. But keep oils refrigerated, and don't cook them long and hot. This makes them oxidize quickly and leads to health problems.

    - *Grains:* Eat whole grains only like plain oatmeal and brown rice. Many people with digestive systems ruined by addictions and some people with mental health diagnoses don't digest grains well. If you crave or have digestive problems, avoid wheat, corn, rye, and oats for a while and stick with the rices.

11. Read labels and root out hydrogenated fats and high fructose corn syrup.

    - The current Suppers recommendation is to avoid *hydrogenated oils, "trans fats," as well as high fructose corn syrup.* They are newcomers to the human diet and implicated in chronic degenerative disease. Some research is showing them to be poisonous in the doses Americans are eating them, leading to chronic degenerative diseases like heart disease, stroke, and diabetes. The products that contain them are not whole foods anyway and are tickets to obesity and diabetes.

These guidelines will be updated as new information is shared at meetings.

Nutritional Protocol to Follow When Eliminating Coffee

These guidelines were prepared by W. George McAuliffe, a certified clinical nutritionist and advisor to The Suppers Programs. Detoxifying is a highly individual matter, sometimes requiring the assistance of a medical nutrition professional. These guidelines are general. Going cold turkey off caffeine can result in about nine days of headache, fatigue, and discomfort. Here is a gentler alternative.

Diet

- Increase the consumption of fiber-rich plant foods (fruits, vegetables, whole grains, legumes, and raw nuts and seeds).

- Increase protein intake (fish, fowl), consume protein every three hours during your waking day.

- Avoid the intake of caffeine, nicotine, other stimulants and alcohol.

- Identify food allergies, avoid these foods.

- Increase consumption of pure water to half your weight in ounces.

Nutritional Supplements

- High potency Multiple Vitamin and Mineral

- Vitamin C: 1000 – 3000 mg 3 times daily

- Vitamin E: 200 – 400 IU daily

- EPA-DHA: 2 capsules 3 times daily

- 5 HTTP: 100 – 200 mg 3 times daily

- Folic Acid and B12: 800 mcg of each daily

Facilitator Dos and Don'ts

How will you know when you are ready to facilitate your own meeting? You may have already co-facilitated another meeting, experienced growth in the program, and articulated your experience in the form of a story that's posted on the Suppers web site. There is nothing that says you need to have all the skills; you can team up and co-facilitate with someone who fills in your blanks, like cooking if you aren't proficient.

Do model "I statements," sharing thoughts, beliefs and personal experiences.

Don't tell them how it is.

Do share your personal experience and experiments.

Don't ever tell someone what to do.

> Suppers is about supporting people's change process. That involves practicing not knowing. To get how this looks, you probably have to have attended enough meetings to have personal experience of the positive effects of acceptance and validation of your competence to choose your own path. This doesn't seem to be human nature, so practicing motivational interviewing skills may be required.

Do suggest readings and resources that may help them find their answers.

Don't promote a particular book or diet.

Do encourage members to take over some of the responsibilities of the meetings such as reading some of the opening, leading the opening and/or a meditation/breathing exercise, encouraging them to give book reports or feedback on something they have learned.

When introducing a controversial topic, don't allow crosstalk or feedback.

Do go once around the table, allowing each person who wants to speak, but not to refute, put down or in any way judge what someone else has shared.

Do not take on the responsibility of knowing everybody's allergies and/or preferences. That is the members' responsibilities.

Do have them participate in the food preparation and make sure their needs are met.

Do share your negative experiences with a particular course of action.

Don't try to bias them against something that didn't work for you but might work for them.

Do encourage them to experiment, as in the Breakfast Challenge, trying exercise such as walking or yoga and observing or journaling the experience.

Do let people know they can contact you at a separate time if they ask you during a meeting about your professional services.

Don't promote your services at meetings.

At meetings where there are people with portion-size issues, do serve the food yourself for everyone.

Don't publicly criticize someone with portion problems.

> Overeating is a very common problem among the people who would be attracted to Suppers. Many of our brains have been hijacked by refined foods. This is Suppers; they don't have the option of paying for two portions. This is where new behaviors are modeled and tried out. It's OK to talk about wanting to buy muffins after a meeting. It's important to be honest about the disappointment people may feel because program food doesn't provide a "hit" of their favorite food drugs.

Do describe the available materials to support change, when they become ready.

Don't advocate any particular course of action.

Do allow sharing about members' own good experiences with doctors or other professionals.

Don't refer. Members can talk about this elsewhere, not at the table/meeting.

Do have clear boundaries and a vetting process (referrals from current members, for example) if you are inviting people into your home.

Don't accept into the group people whom you are uncomfortable having in your home.

> Meetings in private homes are very different from meetings in public settings because on top of the expectations that all members protect the safety of the setting, there are house rules. Although the only requirement for membership is the desire to lead a healthier life, it is a privilege to be invited into your home. Hosts may expect guests to observe house rules.

Do be prepared for members to judge and hold forth. They are only human. Have stock responses ready to ease them back to the Suppers way of being:

> Can you put that into an "I" statement? In other words, can you share that as your point of view, your opinion, or your experience?

> Let me help you get on track. At Suppers, the first concept is biological individuality, which requires each of us to understand our personal biology through self-observation.

> I need to stop you a moment. At Suppers we make an active practice of nonjudgment. Can you state that again without making anyone else's opinion wrong?

> I need to stop you a moment. At Suppers meetings, there are no experts. Can you speak to the personal reasons you want to come to our program?

What Suppers Facilitators Can Apply from the Spirit of Motivational Interviewing

This document on the spirit of motivational interviewing was prepared for Suppers facilitators. The original document by Rollnick and Miller, below, appeared in Behavioral and Cognitive Psychotherapy, 1995. Notes on operating in the spirit of MI for Suppers facilitators are in *italics*.

Introduction

The concept of motivational interviewing evolved from experience in the treatment of problem drinkers, and was first described by Miller (1983) in an article published in Behavioural Psychotherapy. These fundamental concepts and approaches were later elaborated by Miller and Rollnick (1991) in a more detailed description of clinical procedures. A noteworthy omission from both of these documents, however, was a clear definition of motivational interviewing.

We thought it timely to describe our own conceptions of the essential nature of motivational interviewing. Any innovation tends to be diluted and changed with diffusion (Rogers, 1994). Furthermore, some approaches being delivered under the name of motivational interviewing (c.g., Kuchipudi, Hobein, Fleckinger and Iber, 1990) bear little resemblance to our understanding of its essence, and indeed in some cases directly violate what we regard to be central characteristics. For these reasons, we have prepared this description of: (1) a definition of motivational interviewing, (2) a terse account of what we regard to be the essential *spirit* of the approach; (3) differentiation of motivational interviewing from related methods with which it tends to be confused; (4) a brief update on outcome research evaluating its efficacy; and (5) a discussion of new applications that are emerging. *(Link for full document: http://www.motivationalinterview.org/clinical/whatismi.html)*

Definition

Our best current definition is this: **Motivational interviewing is a directive, client-centered counseling style for eliciting behavior change by helping clients to explore and resolve ambivalence.** Compared with non-directive counseling, it is more focused and goal-directed. The examination and resolution of ambivalence is its central purpose, and the counselor is intentionally directive in pursuing this goal.

The Spirit of Motivational Interviewing

Consider how we can operate in this spirit at Suppers.

We believe it is vital to distinguish between the *spirit* of motivational interviewing and *techniques* that we have recommended to manifest that spirit. Clinicians and trainers who become too focused on matters of technique can lose sight of the spirit and style that are central to the approach. There are as many variations in technique as there are clinical encounters. The spirit of the method, however, is move enduring and can be characterized in a few key points.

1. **Motivation to change is elicited from the client, and not imposed from without.** Other motivational approaches have emphasized coercion, persuasion, constructive confrontation, and the use of external contingencies (e.g., the threatened loss of job or family). Such strategies may have their place in evoking change, but they are quite different in spirit from

motivational interviewing, which relies upon identifying and mobilizing the client's intrinsic values and goals to stimulate behaviour change.

An example that comes up often at Suppers is what motivates dietary change for people with type 2 diabetes or other health challenges related to habits of diet and lifestyle. What do you personally need when you are working on change?

2. **It is the client's task, not the counselor's, to articulate and resolve his or her ambivalence.** Ambivalence takes the form of a conflict between two courses of action (e.g., indulgence versus restraint), each of which has perceived benefits and costs associated with it. Many clients have never had the opportunity of expressing the often confusing, contradictory and uniquely personal elements of this conflict, for example, "If I stop smoking I will feel better about myself, but I may also put on weight, which will make me feel unhappy and unattractive." The counsellor's task is to facilitate expression of both sides of the ambivalence impasse, and guide the client toward an acceptable resolution that triggers change.

We can examine this nonjudgmentally using the "once-around-the-table" approach, with no crosstalk or opinions on another's sharing.

3. **Direct persuasion is not an effective method for resolving ambivalence.** It is tempting to try to be "helpful" by persuading the client of the urgency of the problem about the benefits of change. It is fairly clear, however, that these tactics generally increase client resistance and diminish the probability of change (Miller, Benefield and Tonigan, 1993, Miller and Rollnick, 1991).

Let's examine our own inclinations to be urgent about others. Some of us may be able to describe how other's urgency to make us change has worked for us.

4. **The counselling style is generally a quiet and eliciting one.** Direct persuasion, aggressive confrontation, and argumentation are the conceptual opposite of motivational interviewing and are explicitly proscribed in this approach. To a counsellor accustomed to confronting and giving advice, motivational interviewing can appear to be a hopelessly slow and passive process. The proof is in the outcome. More aggressive strategies, sometimes guided by a desire to "confront client denial," easily slip into pushing clients to make changes for which they are not ready.

For facilitators, it may help to consider what happened when someone told us we were in denial or tried to push us into healthier decisions.

5. **The counsellor is directive in helping the client to examine and resolve ambivalence.** Motivational interviewing involves no training of clients in behavioural coping skills, although the two approaches are not incompatible. The operational assumption in motivational interviewing is that ambivalence or lack of resolve is the principal obstacle to be overcome in triggering change. Once that has been accomplished, there may or may not be a need for further intervention such as skill training. The specific strategies of motivational interviewing are designed to elicit, clarify, and resolve ambivalence in a client-centred and respectful counselling atmosphere.

Can anyone share on how the gentle, nonjudgmental environment at Suppers allowed their decisions about change to emerge?

6. **Readiness to change is not a client trait, but a fluctuating product of interpersonal interaction.** The therapist is therefore highly attentive and responsive to the client's

motivational signs. Resistance and "denial" are seen not as client traits, but as feedback regarding therapist behaviour. Client resistance is often a signal that the counsellor is assuming greater readiness to change than is the case, and it is a cue that the therapist needs to modify motivational strategies.

In the case of Suppers facilitators, "resistance" lets us know we need to examine our own methods and motivations. Examples?

7. **The therapeutic relationship is more like a partnership or companionship than expert/recipient roles.** The therapist respects the client's autonomy and freedom of choice (and consequences) regarding his or her own behavior.

   Our version is therapeutic friendship. Share examples of healing that have taken place in the context of Suppers relationships.

Viewed in this way, it is inappropriate to think of motivational interviewing as a technique or set of techniques that are applied to or (worse) "used on" people. Rather, it is an interpersonal style, not at all restricted to formal counseling settings. It is a subtle balance of directive and client-centered components, shaped by a guiding philosophy and understanding of what triggers change. If it becomes a trick or a manipulative technique, its essence has been lost (Miller, 1994).

There are, nevertheless, specific and trainable therapist behaviors that are characteristic of a motivational interviewing style. Foremost among these are:

- Seeking to understand the person's frame of reference, particularly via reflective listening. *We all work on this at meetings, as the active practice of nonjudgment is one of only three absolute requirements of the program. The others being: 1) that our only food bias is that in favor of whole food, and 2) our intolerance of commercial messages or the promotion of particular diets, products, or services.*
- Expressing acceptance and affirmation. *In our case, boundary 7, honoring each other's competence to find our own path to better health.*
- Eliciting and selectively reinforcing the client's own self-motivational statements expressions of problem recognition, concern, desire and intention to change, and ability to change. *Again, evidenced in our requirement to keep the focus on one's self, including the facilitator, and honor each other's competence.*
- Monitoring the client's degree of readiness to change, and ensuring that resistance is not generated by jumping ahead of the client. *In our case, reiterating at each meeting that they receive support regardless of the pace of their progress.*
- Affirming the client's freedom of choice and self-direction. *We operate in this spirit with our first boundary: the only requirement for membership is the desire to lead a healthier life.*

The point is that it is the **spirit** of motivational interviewing that gives rise to these and other specific strategies, and informs their use. A more complete description of the clinical style has been provided by Miller and Rollnick (1991).

Facilitators are invited to notice how, now that you have had this introduction to the model of Motivational Interviewing, you see the spirit of MI at work in our program design and the environment of our meetings.

Opening

Let gratitude fill me,
Family and friendship sustain me
And respect for my body, mind and spirit
Guide my choices.

Closing

Thank you for joining
Our family table,
For offering your friendship
And sharing your self.
Our parting wish for you
Is that you find
The healthier life you seek
In body, mind, and spirit.

Please Get Comfortable Washing Your Hands and Asking Others to Wash Theirs

We ask that you wash your hands:

1. After handling money and before handling food.

2. After you cough into your hand.

3. After touching your face.

We welcome many people with special concerns about their immune systems. We encourage you to help us maintain the standards about hand washing.

Please stay home if you're coughing.

Please do cough into your shoulder.

Please feel free to touch elbows instead of holding hands during the opening and closing.

Three Principles

For the sake of healing for the greatest number, please join us in observing these principles:

1. Actively practice nonjudgment. Offer no advice. Tolerate no criticism.

2. Embrace whole food.
    At meetings, you'll find no gluten or sugar, and very limited dairy and processed food.

3. Be free of commercial messages. Avoid promotion of any particular diet, product or service.

Qualifying for Suppers Facilitation

The heart and soul of Suppers are the facilitators who volunteer their time because they are passionate about sharing what they know.

The program is transmitted member-to-member at meetings and through our literature. So it is important for facilitators to be well versed in the principles, boundaries and concepts at the core of our program design.

To become a qualified facilitator, the training includes:

1. Reading <u>Logical Miracles</u>

2. Writing responses to the book that demonstrate you have internalized key points

3. Attending facilitator training sessions that include:
   - Beginner workshop with groceries
   - Blood sugar and mood chemistry stabilization
   - How you feel is *data*
   - Principles, boundaries and concepts
   - Running a personal inventory meeting
   - Nutritional harm reduction
   - Motivational Interviewing and Stages of Change
   - Getting your needs met (include Nonviolent Communication)

4. And may additionally include:
   - Healthy sources of flavor
   - Knife skills and kitchen hygiene
   - How to set up journals (like food/mood, seasonal, art therapy)
   - Experiments, including breakfast challenge. Includes helping people track progress and share results at meetings
   - Preparing for change/setting good goals, for people who don't know how to set up doable goals (good for self-saboteurs)
   - Stress reduction
   - Meditations
   - Developing your Suppers story to share and post
   - Book reviews
   - Planning is everything
   - Palate development
   - Digestion
   - Fats and oils
   - Acid and alkaline foods

5. Run a meeting with a qualified facilitator who will remain in the co-facilitator role (from planning the menu to buying groceries, set up food prep, select topic and reading and leading the meeting).

6. Read and present on a book that has inspired you, and model I statements and non-judgment while presenting.

7. Submit two recipes formatted on our template for posting.

Types of Qualification

Qualified Facilitator: You have completed the training and run your own at least monthly meeting, minimum ten per year.

Qualified Co-facilitator: You have completed the facilitator training and you co-facilitate a regular meeting, at least monthly, minimum ten per year.

Guest Facilitator: You host at least four special meetings per year with a co-facilitator helping.

Facilitator Trainee: You are in the process and have articulated the kind of meeting you want to run and set a starting date.

Recognition will take place at the regularly scheduled facilitator meetings; and meetings may of course celebrate their facilitators.

<u>Logical Miracles</u> Written Responses

Select a reading with which you identify and write a paragraph or two about how it is relevant for you.

Describe in a paragraph or two how you would handle this situation: You sense the beginnings of an argument among people with differing views on a subject (example, how much protein a person should eat, or the best way to lose weight, or a point of parenting). Set up your scenario and tell how you would put the meeting back on track, referring to the principles, boundaries and concepts that guide us.

Script a one-minute meditation or breathing exercise that you would use before saying the opening to help people quiet down, get in touch with their bodies, and prepare for the meal.

At large meetings or where a meeting is challenging to control, we gather people to the purpose of Suppers by going once around the table and allowing each person to share with no commenting or cross talk. The subject of the meeting is "How you feel is *data*." Set up your scenario and script how you will get this meeting on track, using the once-around-the-table approach.

The spiritual foundation of Suppers is the notion that caring for the body is the primary spiritual act because the body is the temple of the soul. How do you relate to this notion?

Suppers is about progress not perfection. In a paragraph or two, describe your understanding of nutritional harm reduction and give examples of how you have reduced harm nutritionally yourself.

Explain the importance of distinguishing treats from triggers and in a paragraph or two give an example in your personal experience.

Describe the population you would like to serve at Suppers and what motivates you to do this.

Service Club

Facilitators have the option of joining the service club and logging your hours.

- Four hours for each meeting you facilitate
- Two hours for each meeting you co-facilitate
- For training you get the number of approved hours for that event
- For any relevant other training (Non-program, like cooking classes, lectures on healthy living, workshops related to the theme of your meeting) you receive Continuing Education (CE) credit

Credit for CE hours may not exceed your total facilitator and co-facilitator hours.

Bonus hours: For each new meeting you help launch (so, meetings that are less than three months old), you get double hours.

Name:			
Checklist for Facilitator Qualification			
Date	**Approved**	**Task**	**Comments**
		Read <u>Logical Miracles</u>	
		Submit response to questions on <u>Logical Miracles</u>	
		Attend facilitator training sessions on: • Beginner workshop	
		• Blood sugar and mood chemistry stabilization	
		• How you feel is data	
		• Principles, boundaries and concepts	
		• Running a personal inventory meeting	
		• Nutritional harm reduction	
		• Motivational interviewing and stages of change	
		• Getting your needs met	
		• Other training session(s)	Other topic -
		Run a meeting with a qualified facilitator	
		Submit two ready-to-post recipes on Suppers template	
		Read and present on a book that has inspired you, and model "I" statements and non-judgment while presenting	
		Register as a qualified facilitator on the Suppers web site	
		Start recording your hours!	

Mission

The Suppers mission is to provide safe and friendly settings where anyone – and especially people with food-related health challenges – can develop and manage their own personal transitions to a healthier life.

Four principles guide us in our mission:

1. The active practice of nonjudgement
2. Whole food preparation
3. No commercial messages
4. Restoration of the family table

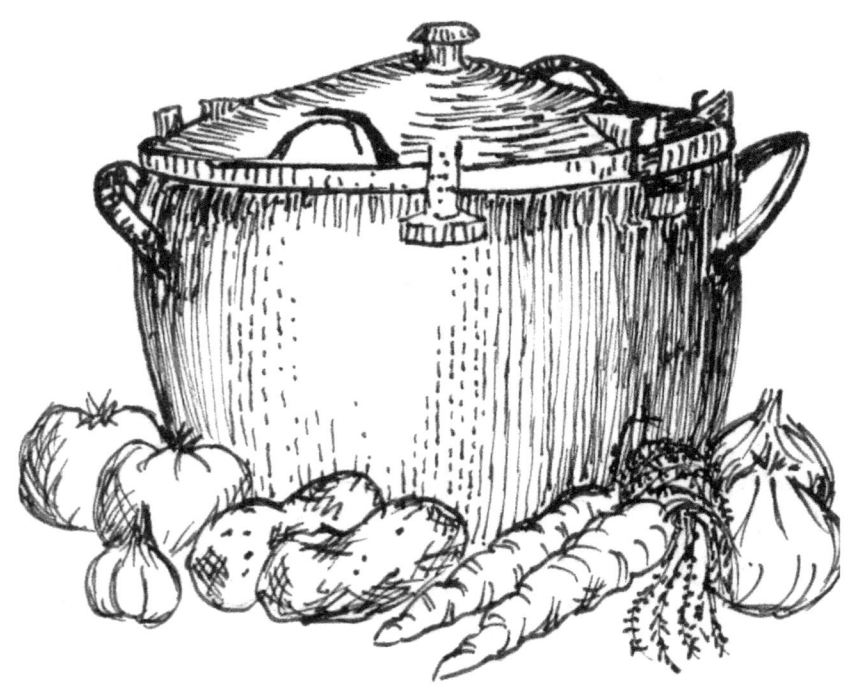

"If you can make a pot of coffee, you can make a pot of soup."

There are as many kinds of Suppers groups as there are people who are willing to share their gifts with others who want to lead a healthier life. For information about starting your own Suppers meeting, please contact us at Dor@TheSuppersPrograms.org.

For more recipes and members' stories, visit www.TheSuppersPrograms.org.

www.ingramcontent.com/pod-product-compliance
Lightning Source LLC
Chambersburg PA
CBHW082143290526
45794CB00008B/3142